D0882272

DR. MOYAD'S

No BS

~~Diet~~

Health Advice

Mark Moyad, MD, MPH

All inquiries should be addressed to:
Spry Publishing
2500 S. State St.
Ann Arbor, MI 48104
Phone 877-722-2264

Manufactured in the United States of America
by Edwards Brothers, Inc.

ISBN 13: 978-1-58726-256-2
ISBN 10: 1-58726-256-8

10 9 8 7 6 5 4 3

Disclaimer: Spry Publishing does not assume responsibility for the contents or opinions expressed herein. Although every precaution is taken to ensure that information is accurate as of the date of publication, differences of opinion exist. The opinions in this document are those of the author and do not necessarily reflect the views of the publisher. All information contained in this document should be discussed with the patient's doctor prior to beginning or changing the patient's course of treatment.

To my parents (Robert aka Dad and Eva aka Mom) and brothers (Andy and Tom), who were simply the best parents and brothers a kid could have.

To my mentors/bosses at the University of Michigan (Dr. Bloom, Dr. Montie, and Dr. Pienta) for always supporting and believing in me.

To the donors of my endowment (Jenkins, Pokempner, Thompson, and Epstein) for helping to make this world a better place one starfish at a time.

To my wife, Mia, and my stepdaughter and stepson, Holly and Nick, who really made me the luckiest man in the world!

Finally, to my big sister Tawn and to my cousin Firouzeh, you simply deserved better, but we will at least make sure that people know and learn from your situation.

Mia, my wife, I appreciate you never throwing me outside with the dog while I was writing this book during our vacations! However, sleeping in the bathtub was difficult, and I think I hurt my back!

Contents

Preface

Hey, can you smell it? The smell of B.S. when it comes to health advice—yes, the smell of B.S. or "Bogus Science." I can, because it stinks so badly I can hardly breathe anymore! Come in closer and look, because you have smelled it for years, but you did not know what it was and exactly from where it came. I smelled it for about twenty years and have been telling thousands of doctors and other health-care workers and individuals around the world about this smell and how to avoid it!

Hi, I'm Dr. Moyad (I sound like a bad commercial but, hey, give me some credit because I am passionate and like to keep it personal). Occupying an endowed position as the Jenkins/Pokempner Director of Preventive and Alternative Medicine, Department of Urology, University of Michigan Medical Center, created and funded entirely by patients, allows me to be refreshingly objective and candid about what works and what is worthless to stay healthy.

You have been asked to buy into all the health advice for years—by buying books, the machines, the newsletters, the pills, the injections, the surgeries—but now it is time to put these to rest for a while and empower yourself with the knowledge to sort through all the B.S. So let's begin!

INTRODUCTION
Heart Healthy = All Healthy

The Perfect Realistic, Practical &
Probability-Based Partnership

We all seem to live our lives on probability, except when it comes to our health. For example, there are no guarantees, but probability is why we board a plane, wear a seatbelt, get an education, have a baby, and even get married.

So, why don't we follow probability or learn from probability when it comes to our health? I see women and men all the time who are concerned about breast or prostate cancer, but who cannot tell me their cholesterol and blood pressure numbers. This is not only scary but also ignores the probability of what could really get them in the blink of an eye or, to be more candid, kill them in a moment! I also meet people all the time who know their cholesterol numbers, but who have never had a flu shot or a colonoscopy.

Let's focus on your health and probability for a moment. Take a look at the list of the top six killers of women and men, and what you may notice is that the only real difference between women and men in terms of causes of death is that Alzheimer's disease is now one of the top causes of death in women. However, this is the result of a population that is living longer compared to any generation before it. Women on average live five to eight years longer than men (personally, I do not think this is fair), and aging or just living a long life is one of the most common risk factors for this disease. Therefore, as the life expectancy of men increases, Alzheimer's disease is expected to be one of the top causes of death for both sexes.

Top 6 Killers of Women

1. Cardiovascular disease (CVD)
2. Cancer (lung, breast, colon)
3. Respiratory/Lung disease
4. Alzheimer's disease
5. Diabetes
6. Pneumonia/Flu

Top 6 Killers of Men

1. Cardiovascular disease (CVD)
2. Cancer (lung, prostate, colon)
3. Accidents (automobile …)
4. Respiratory/Lung disease
5. Diabetes
6. Pneumonia/Flu

What we can learn from this list is that improving heart health is your best chance of living longer and better. The heart-healthy diet is the exact same one that is touted to prevent all the other common causes of death in the list. For example, if you look at the latest information on preventing cancer, Alzheimer's, or diabetes, the lifestyle recommendations are exactly the same as the heart-healthy recommendations (lower weight and blood pressure, exercise …)—they are just repackaged and sold as an anticancer or anti-diabetes or an Alzheimer's prevention diet.

I'm often asked how many different things in life can affect or boost your immune system? The answer might surprise you! So many behaviors, conditions, and products influence your immune health that it is almost frightening. The good news is that many of the things that affect your immune health are behaviors that are in your control, which should put your mind at ease and encourage you to take even more control of your health and wellness. Just a partial listing of both the items in your control and those that are not is given in the table.

Factors That Affect Your Immune System (and Overall Health)	Comment
Age	Older (or a more politically correct term is chronologically advantaged or seasoned) and very young individuals are more likely to have a weaker immune system, as are individuals with chronic diseases.
Alcohol	Moderate to even slightly higher levels of alcohol intake from any source (beer, wine, hard liquor) on a regular basis can reduce the effectiveness of your immune system.

Blood pressure/ Cholesterol	High blood pressure and/or high cholesterol levels may lead to immune problems that may cause heart disease to become worse.
Dental disease	An unhealthy mouth can cause bacteria to travel to other body sites, causing your immune system to work overtime.
Diabetes and other diseases	High glucose (sugar) and other abnormal numbers indicate conditions that compromise your immune defenses.
Diet	Heart-healthy diets are immune healthy, but that also means that heart-unhealthy diets are immune-unhealthy diets.
Environment (in and outside the home)	Exposure to all types of pollution is bad for your immune system.
Genetics/Family history	Immune problems can also run in families, such as allergies and asthma.
Infections and illnesses	A minor or major infection can cause problems.
Medical procedures	Contrast agents, excessive amounts of radiation, and other compounds used for certain medical procedures all have implications for your immune system.
Mental health	Depression, for example, can decrease immune function, whereas laughter can boost immunity.
Menstrual cycle/Hormone changes (in women and men)	Nutritional fluctuations and needs occur at these times, for example, with calcium and vitamin C, and this includes men losing testosterone over time.
Medications (prescriptions and dietary supplements)	Steroids and other pills work by suppressing the immune response, but this may come at the price of a weakened immune system. However, other drugs and supplements may strengthen the immune system, such as those that are heart healthy.
Physical activity	Moderate exercise is healthy, but extreme exercise or no exercise can cause immune suppression.

Factors That Affect Your Immune System (and Overall Health)	Comment
Pregnancy	All trimesters of pregnancy cause immune changes, which is why pregnancy is the most critical time in life to be immune healthy. Increased attention is being focused on getting more vitamin D and omega-3 fatty acids during this time.
Sleep	Reduced sleep by even a few hours a night can be immune suppressive.
Smoke (smokers or secondhand smoke)	Smoking leads to nutrient decreases in the blood, which also leads to immune dysfunction. Even secondhand smoke can cause immune problems.
Stress (physical or mental)	Hormones are released with stress and work like steroids to suppress the immune system.
Temperature changes	Extreme warmth and cold are not good for your immune health.
Weight	Higher weight, body mass index, and, especially, greater waist circumference can lead to a weak immune system.

Again, heart disease or, more accurately, cardiovascular disease (CVD), is the number-one killer of women and men. In general, what research has shown to be heart healthy has also turned out to be immune healthy.

Cardiovascular disease actually kills more women than men now, and this has been the case since 1984! Therefore, since CVD is the number-one cause of death in women and men, if you become more heart healthy you may get a "2 for 1" effect, so to speak. Think about this for a second—our real health goal is not just to live longer but also to live better with a higher quality of life. The only real way to achieve this goal is simply to improve your chances or your probability of living longer and better by following many lifestyle changes that impact your immune system and the most common diseases, not just one disease.

So, before we continue, let's review the words I like to repeat to patients and myself every day:

HEART HEALTHY = Anti-Aging Healthy = Bladder Healthy = Bone Healthy = Brain Healthy = Breast Healthy = Colon Healthy = Dental Healthy = Eye Healthy = Immune Healthy = Joint & Muscle Healthy = Kidney Healthy = Mental Health = Orgasm/Reproductive/Sexual Healthy = Prostate Healthy = Skin Healthy = ALL HEALTHY

If you are following a real heart-healthy diet, then you are following the best diet possible to reduce your risk of disease and early death, not only now but in the future. Now, my friends, buckle your seatbelts because we are about to have a lot of fun and learn a lot at the same time.

Mark A. Moyad, MD, MPH
Jenkins/Pokempner Director of
Preventive & Alternative Medicine
University of Michigan Medical Center
Department of Urology

Part I

Dr. Moyad's No B.S. Risk Assessment

There are ten not-so-easy steps to measure your risk for what has the highest probability of killing you. That does not sound politically correct ... for those offended by the word "killing," insert the words "eliminating my pulse forever" or "officially relieving me of ever paying taxes again" or "ensuring that there will be no more future conversations with any telemarketers."

Please remember: Heart Healthy = All Healthy, and Heart Unhealthy = All Unhealthy! Repeat this No Bogus Science saying at least once a day for better mental and physical health when you hear conflicting information from the so-called Dr. B.S. "experts."

| Dr. B.S.

"You should worry about getting cancer; now that is a bad disease."

| Dr. Moyad's No B.S.

"Whatever! It has never made sense to me for you to try to remove yourself from the path of an oncoming truck, only to potentially walk in front of an oncoming car. In other words, reducing your risk of the number-one (cardiovascular disease) and number-two (cancer) causes of death is far better than reducing your risk of one or the other. So, you need to follow a plan that helps you reduce your risk of the most common diseases, but in the end heart healthy rules because it is all healthy."

Preventive medicine needs to be triaged, which means it has to be prioritized into what can kill me overnight, realistically speaking of course, to what diseases can kill me overnight or over the next several years or over the next several decades. So, let's triage or prioritize your risk right now in this section and make sure first and foremost that we are living the Heart Healthy = All Healthy way of life.

Before we begin, let's quickly test your health knowledge and do a quick fill-in-the-blank six-question quiz.

1. Yesterday I turned on the TV and watched one of my favorite programs in the world called the *Oprah* _____ *Show*, and then in the evening I like to watch the *Larry* _____ *Show* on CNN, and late at night I like to watch either Jay _____ or David _____ or Conan _____ because they also have great guests.

2. My last vitamin D blood test, which could play a critical part in preventing me from having or dying from a bone fracture, was _____ ng/ml or nmol/L, and I know that the normal number for me on this test is _____ ng/ml or nmol/L.

3. Brad Pitt is married to Angelina _____.

4. My last LDL cholesterol level that can help determine if I may be alive in the next year was _____ mg/dL or mmol/L, and I know that the normal number for me on this test is _____ mg/dL or mmol/L.

5. Paris _____ seems to get a lot of TV time; Denzel _____ is a good actor; and _____ Trump owns a lot of real estate and is on TV a lot.

6. My Framingham Risk Score or Reynolds Risk Score, which can potentially predict whether or not I should take aspirin or whether or not I might live or die in the next ten years, is ____ points, which translates to a ____ percent risk of heart disease.

My total score ____ (Each full question correctly answered gives you one point.)

(Be honest! If you got questions 1, 3, and 5 right and left 2, 4, or 6 blank, you are like everyone else. If you answered only questions 2, 4, and 6, you are a nerd and need to get a social life. If you were able to answer all the questions, you decided, like I did, to wake up and write a book filled with good lifesaving information, along with ridiculous, silly, and mindless observations.)

Part I of this book contains steps to guide you in a health-risk assessment. Some individuals simply will need an executive physical, and others will need an overall heath physical at your nearest medical center to get the answers. Each step you take in this section will move you farther and farther from the big pile of Bogus Science. You will notice that, as you move farther from it, you might feel healthier, both mentally and physically.

Step 1 around the B.S.—Fasting Cholesterol Test

| Dr. B.S.

"All you need is a basic total cholesterol test."

| Dr. Moyad's No B.S.

"Whatever! Just getting a total cholesterol test is like getting the smallest single piece of a puzzle that contains hundreds of pieces. In other words, you need a full cholesterol panel to really get some idea of what your health puzzle looks like right now."

So, let's explore what a cholesterol test involves. The blood test is usually done after fasting for 9 to 12 hours and measures four things—total cholesterol, LDL (bad cholesterol), HDL (good cholesterol), and triglycerides. Those items are worth some definition to help you understand their importance.

Total Cholesterol: an overview number developed using the Friedewald formula, which states that:

$$\text{Total cholesterol} = \text{LDL} + \text{HDL} + (\text{triglycerides} \div 5)$$

Low-density lipoproteins (LDL): LDL, also called "bad" cholesterol, can cause buildup of plaque on the walls of arteries. The more LDL there is in the blood, the greater the risk of heart disease.

High-density lipoproteins (HDL): HDL, also called "good" cholesterol, helps the body get rid of bad cholesterol in the blood. The higher the level of HDL cholesterol, the better. If your levels of HDL are low, your risk of heart disease increases.

Triglycerides: Triglycerides are a type of fat that is carried in the blood. Excess calories in the body are converted into triglycerides and stored in fat cells throughout the body.

Cholesterol numbers are measured in mg/dL (milligrams per deciliter) in the United States and mmol/L (millimoles per liter) in other countries. The following table provides information on understanding your cholesterol scores:

Cholesterol Type	Dr. Moyad's No B.S. Commentary
Total Cholesterol	**Lower is better.**
<160 mg/dL (<4.1 mmol/L)	Ideal or optimal
160–200 mg/dL (4.14–5.16 mmol/L)	Desirable or not bad
200–239 mg/dL (5.16–6.19 mmol/L)	Borderline high
≥240 mg/dL (≥6.22 mmol/L)	High
LDL ("Bad cholesterol")	**Lower is better.**
<70 mg/dL (<1.81 mmol/L)	May be ideal for some high-risk individuals (those who have already experienced a cardiovascular event or are considered "high risk" for a cardiovascular event). However, 10 years from now this may be the new normal level. Personally, I believe everyone should try to achieve this level.
<100 mg/dL (<2.59 mmol/L)	Ideal or optimal for most individuals (Dr. Moyad thinks everyone should have an LDL less than 100 right now.)
100–129 mg/dL (2.59–3.34 mmol/L)	Near ideal or optimal/above optimal (feels better … almost there)
130–159 mg/dL (3.37–4.12 mmol/L)	Borderline high (I do not like this number.)
160–189 mg/dL (4.14–4.90 mmol/L)	High (Fix this problem now.)
≥190 mg/dL (≥4.92 mmol/L)	Very high (Fix this problem immediately.)
HDL ("Good cholesterol")	**Higher is better.** (just like your kids' grades)
≥60 mg/dL (≥1.55 mmol/L)	High or ideal (Awesome or A+)
40–59 mg/dL (1.04–1.53 mmol/L)	Less than ideal (but normal … not bad)
<40 mg/dL (<1.04 mmol/L)	Too low (not good—needs work ASAP)

Triglycerides (fat in the blood)	Lower is better.
<100 mg/dL (<1.13 mmol/L)	Dr. Moyad thinks everyone, especially women, should be below 100!
101–149 mg/dL (1.13–1.69 mmol/L)	Normal (I guess)
150–199 mg/dL (1.70–2.25 mmol/L)	Borderline high (reduce this ASAP)
200–499 mg/dL (2.26–5.64 mmol/L)	High (reduce this now)
≥500 mg/dL (≥5.65 mmol/L)	Too high (Do I need to say anything else?)

Ideally, a fasting cholesterol level should contain all the different types of cholesterol. If a non-fasting cholesterol level is taken, then only the total cholesterol and HDL cholesterol levels are considered partially accurate, and the LDL and triglyceride levels cannot be accurately determined in many cases. Come on, let's cut to the chase and just fast before your next cholesterol test. If you do not fast and your cholesterol numbers are high, then you will usually be asked to fast and repeat this test, and who has time for all this B.S.?

Why is the cholesterol blood test, like any other blood test, not perfect; or, why do some people with low cholesterol have heart attacks?

Cholesterol testing is a wonderful way to get a basic idea of how you are doing. Although it is one of our best tests, there is one sobering fact about the limitations of this test. *Approximately half of the women and men that suffer a first-time heart attack have a normal cholesterol level!* Additional research suggests some other blood tests may help to predict your risk along with cholesterol testing. You should know about some of them because your doctor may want to use them, or you may find it unacceptable that they are not being discussed or used on you. See Step 2 for a list of the tests.

Your Goal: Have your cholesterol levels checked after a 9–12-hour fast (going without food and beverages, except plain old water), and compare your results with the ranges in the table.

Step 2 around the B.S.—Blood Tests

Ask your doctor about other blood tests (placed in alphabetical order—not in the order of importance) that may determine your cardiovascular risk or that may enhance the results of your cholesterol test. *Cardiovascular disease kills more women than men every year*, but in the majority of surveys almost two-thirds of women asked do not know what an HDL or LDL is or what their specific level is, and men do not do any better in these surveys. Whether or not you get any or all of these tests should be discussed with your physician.

| Dr. B.S.

"The only important blood test for heart disease risk is a fasting cholesterol panel that tells you your total cholesterol, HDL, LDL, and triglycerides."

| Dr. Moyad's No B.S.

"You have to ask your doctor about other possible blood tests that can further define your cardiovascular risk."

Other Cholesterol or Heart Disease Blood Tests	Dr. Moyad's No B.S. Comments
Apo A (Apolipoprotein A-1)	Numbers should increase with your HDL; if they do not, I become more concerned. Higher numbers are better, indicating a reduced risk, as this test is an estimation of heart-protective particles. Whether or not it predicts risk any better than HDL is controversial.
Apo B (Apolipoprotein B-100)	Numbers should decrease with your LDL; if they do not, I become more concerned. Lower numbers are better! Higher levels may indicate an increased risk, as this test is an estimation of heart disease–promoting particles. Whether or not it predicts risk any better than LDL or non-HDL numbers is controversial.

Cholesterol ratio For example, the total cholesterol/HDL	Lower ratio = lower risk when it comes to total cholesterol/HDL ratio.
HDL subspecies or subtypes (HDL type 2 or HDL type 3)	Higher levels or ratios of HDL 2 to HDL 3 may indicate a reduced risk, as this test is an estimation of heart protective particles. HDL 2 is larger and thought to be more protective, while HDL 3 is smaller and may be less protective. Whether or not it predicts risk any better than HDL is controversial.
LDL or HDL particle size	Higher levels of small LDL or HDL particles may indicate an increased risk, just as higher levels of large LDL or HDL particles may indicate a reduced risk. Whether or not it predicts risk any better than just LDL or HDL is controversial. Also, if your triglyceride level is less than 100 or 150 (normal) and the rest of your basic cholesterol test is normal, many experts think the particle size test is not useful because most particles are not small or not a concern.
Lipoprotein (a) = Lp (a)	Some experts believe that higher levels of Lp (a) may be associated with a higher risk for CVD, especially in men. Whether or not it is any better than knowing your LDL is controversial.
Non-HDL level	Higher levels may be associated with a higher risk. You simply arrive at this number by adding LDL + triglycerides.
Other Tests That Are Important to Your Overall Health	**Dr. Moyad's No B.S. Comments**
Complete blood profile (CBC) and complete metabolic profile	Series of overall health numbers that generally look at your blood cells/counts, anemia risk, sugar levels (glucose), liver function … and should be part of every annual physical exam.

Other Tests That Are Important to Your Overall Health	Dr. Moyad's No B.S. Comments
Glucose (fasting)	Higher levels may be associated with a higher risk (some doctors also get an insulin level with this test). *I like this test for everyone*, and it is usually a part of the complete metabolic profile.
Hemoglobin A1c (also known as "HgbA1c")	This test gives an idea of long-term glucose or sugar levels in the body. Reported as a percentage, in general the lower the percentage the better (some say 6% or 7%, but I say you are competing with yourself). Many diabetics are familiar with this test, but some doctors think non-diabetics should get this test also.
hs-CRP (high-sensitivity C-reactive protein) a measure of low-grade inflammation that may be occurring in your cardiovascular system. There are other inflammatory markers, but these should be discussed with your doctor.	Higher levels may be associated with a higher risk. Some doctors like this test because it is cheap and it has received preliminary testing in women as well as men. *I love this test for everyone!* (especially when the result is below 1). Do not confuse this test with a basic CRP test (without the letters *hs* in front of it), because the basic CRP test is not as sensitive.
Homocysteine	You may have high levels of homocysteine when cholesterol, white blood cells, calcium, and other substances (plaque) build up in your blood vessels. Lower levels may indicate lower risk. Moderate levels of antioxidant vitamins such as B6, B12, and especially folic acid may reduce high levels, but high amounts of these vitamins should not be taken without your doctor's approval. *I like this test* done once in a while because it can catch those individuals with abnormally high levels!

Male & Female Hormone Levels (Note: Some men will need both gender hormones tested as well as some women. For example, it is not unusual to get estradiol and testosterone levels in women with female sexual dysfunction.)	Lower levels can have a negative impact on overall health, but they are easily treated by lifestyle change and/or medication. Men need to have their testosterone taken early in the morning to ensure the accuracy of the test!
Thrombogenic Factor Tests (test for factors causing or resulting in thrombosis or coagulation of the blood)	Lower levels may indicate lower risk—discuss these with your doctor. For example, fibrinogen is the major coagulation protein in blood (it is the precursor to fibrin involved in clotting) and impacts blood thickness. Every increase in fibrinogen by 1 point may be associated with an increased risk of problems, but this is still controversial.
Thyroid Hormone Test (TSH)	This test can tell you if you are making too much, too little, or enough of the thyroid hormone that can control everything from your heart rate to your mental health.
Vitamin D Blood Test (25-OH Vitamin D Test)	This test should be done once a year in the fall or winter for *everyone*. The normal Moyad level should be 35–40 ng/ml or 90–100 nmol/L.
Vitamin C Blood Test and/or Omega Index Text	These are very controversial tests. In some of the largest disease prevention trials, the men and women who had the lowest risk of numerous diseases had higher blood levels of vitamin C and/or omega 3! These just may be good blood markers or indicators of general health!

What if my cholesterol ratios (total cholesterol/HDL, for example) are perfect or outstanding because my HDL is high and my triglycerides are low, but my LDL by itself is still high? My doctor says not to worry about it. What do you think, Dr. Moyad?

I am asked this question by a woman or man at least once every lecture anywhere in the world. HDL works best as a cleaning agent for your body when the LDL is low, so *I do not like a high LDL in any woman or man, even if their ratios are perfect.*

What about coronary calcium scoring using a CT scan (or EBT scan)?

This procedure takes a picture of your heart and the vessels that feed and leave from it. Apparently, the higher the amount of calcium, the greater your risk of a future cardiovascular event. The problem is that these tests are backed by limited research, and they come with a good deal of radiation exposure. Most people need to know everything about their blood tests and risk factors before even thinking about the calcium-scoring test. So, first get an honest assessment of your situation before you decide to pursue options that are supported by less evidence.

Your Goal: Discuss with your doctor what other tests will give a more comprehensive picture of your heart health, especially if you have a strong personal or family history of heart disease.

Step 3 around the B.S.—Blood Pressure

| Dr. B.S.

"High blood pressure kills, so get your blood pressure measured at your doctor's office every time you have a physical exam."

| Dr. Moyad's No B.S.

"Whatever! High blood pressure kills. If I ask you just once a year for three seconds how you are doing and you say just fine, or horrible, or whatever, should I accept this as fact? In other words, is this how you will feel and respond the other 364 days of the year?"

You go to your doctor about once a year maybe and she/he takes one or two blood pressure readings, and that is supposed to define how you are doing for the entire year! Also, keep in mind that high blood pressure is becoming the number-one cause of cardiovascular death around the world! This number is too important, so let's treat it that way. Take a few readings every month or two, record these on a piece of paper, and give that paper to your doctor on every visit! Now, let's figure out what risk category you belong in right now! Blood pressure: you need three separate readings from your doctor's office and, ideally, from home.

| Dr. B.S.

"140 over 90 is a high blood pressure!"

| Dr. Moyad's No B.S.

"Whatever! You need to figure out exactly where you are and what you can do about it. Get a clear picture of your true number because pre-hypertension is also an abnormal number!"

Blood Pressure (systolic/ diastolic)	What does this mean, Dr. Moyad?
<120/80 mmHg	Normal = low risk.
120–139/80–89 mmHg	Pre-hypertensive (moderately high or pre–high blood pressure) = moderate risk.
≥140/90 mmHg	Hypertensive (high blood pressure) = high risk.

The problem with getting an accurate blood pressure reading from your doctor is that some individuals get *white-coat hypertension* (falsely elevated blood pressure in a doctor's office but not at home). White-coat hypertension is medically defined as an office blood pressure of at least 140/90 mmHg, but a daytime reading out of office or at home of less than 135/85 mmHg. Patients with white-coat hypertension are *not* at a higher risk of a cardiovascular event compared to patients with normal blood pressure. Patients with *masked hypertension* (defined as low blood pressure in the doctor's office but high blood pressure at home) or *sustained hypertension* (defined as high blood pressure both in the doctor's office and at home) are at a higher risk of a cardiovascular event compared to individuals with normal blood pressure.

Your Goal: Buy your own automated blood pressure reading machine and use it at home, taking your blood pressure a few times each month. Record the readings and take with you to your next doctor's appointment. Note: *Consumer Reports* magazine, healthcare professionals, medical supply stores, and pharmacies can guide you to find a reliable upper-arm machine that costs less than $100 (if you can, avoid wrist cuff device).

Step 4 around the B.S.—Heart Rate

| **Dr. B.S.**

"Just golf or garden because that is good exercise for your heart!"

| **Dr. Moyad's No B.S.**

"Whatever! Hey, nothing against golf or gardening, but there are times you have to use it or lose it! In other words, the heart is a muscle that should get a workout on a regular basis. This will also improve your mental health, so talk to your doctor about more moderate-to-intense exercise or an exercise that can eventually lower your resting heart rate."

The bottom line is that, in general, the lower your resting heart rate the better (you are only competing against yourself here). Lower heart rates tend to mean that the heart itself is doing less work per beat to pass blood through your body. It is doing less work because the heart muscle itself has become stronger, and this improves your chances of living longer and better. Apparently, Lance Armstrong had (or still has, hopefully) a resting heart rate in the thirties (no surprise)! Most of the longest-living mammals or animals have low resting heart rates, and most of the shortest-living mammals have very high resting heart rates (for example, the mouse). Making your heart rate increase to a higher level during exercise helps to strengthen your heart and lowers your resting heart rate. *However, never ever begin a strenuous exercise program until you get your doctor's approval.*

Your Goal: Record your resting heart rate or pulse several times every few months, and also record your heart rate during or right after moderate-to-intense exercise. Bring these numbers into your doctor on your next visit.

Step 5 around the B.S.—Coronary Heart Disease Risk

| Dr. B.S.

"Risk assessment is difficult for patients, and you need a licensed and experienced physician to first help patients calculate and then understand their risk."

| Dr. Moyad's No B.S.

"Whatever! The main risk assessment tools such as the Framingham Risk Score or the Reynolds Risk Score are so simple, everyone should be taught how to use them."

After you calculate your coronary heart disease (CHD) risk using the information on the next few pages (there are separate sections for men and women), please come back to this table and circle or write in your number.

10-Year Risk of Heart Disease	Comments (Dr. Moyad's quirky banter in parentheses—not meant to be taken seriously.)
>20%	High risk (Stay away from ice cream!)
10–20%	Moderate risk (Ice cream sounds good sometime this month.)
<10%	Low risk (Let's go get ice cream this week.)
<5%	Dr. Moyad low-risk (Yeah! Let's go get some ice cream right now!)

For Women Only

Ladies first ... and this decision is based on the embarrassing track record medicine has for putting cardiovascular risk in women second to that in men.

Calculating Your 10-Year Risk of Heart Disease for Women (also called the Framingham risk score)

A. Find your age group and point value and circle it.

Age (years)	Points
20–34	−7
35–39	−3
40–44	0
45–49	3
50–54	6
55–59	8
60–64	10
65–69	12
70–74	14
75+	16

B. Find your total cholesterol level and match it to your age group, then determine your point value and circle it.

Total Cholesterol (mg/dL or mmol/L)	Age 20–39	Age 40–49	Age 50–59	Age 60–69	Age 70–79
<160 or 4.14	0	0	0	0	0
160–199 or 4.15–5.16	4	3	2	1	1
200–239 or 5.18–6.19	8	6	4	2	1
240–279 or 6.22–7.23	11	8	5	3	2
≥280 or 7.25	13	10	7	4	2

C. Whether you are a current smoker or not, find your age group, and then find your point value and circle it.

Smoking Status Currently	Age 20–39	Age 40–49	Age 50–59	Age 60–69	Age 70–79
Nonsmoker	0	0	0	0	0
Smoker	9	7	4	2	1

D. Locate your HDL number and point value, and circle the point value.

HDL (mg/dL or mmol/L)	Points
≥60 or 1.56	−1
50–59 or 1.3–1.53	0
40–49 or 1.04–1.27	1
<40 or 1.04	2

E. Locate your systolic blood pressure, treated or untreated by medication, and find your point value and circle it.

Systolic BP (mmHg)	Untreated	Treated
<120	0	0
120–129	1	3
130–139	2	4
140–159	3	5
≥160	4	6

F. Add your points from A through E.

Age   Points =

Total cholesterol   Points =

Smoker/nonsmoker   Points =

HDL   Points =

Systolic blood pressure   Points =

Total points   _____

G. Match your total points from F to the table below, circle your 10-year risk of CHD, and bring it to your doctor on your next visit.

Total Points	10-Year Risk
<9	<1%
9–12	1%
13–14	2%
15	3%

16	4%
17	5%
18	6%
19	8%
20	11%
21	14%
22	17%
23	22%
24	27%
≥25	≥30%

For women who have had a recent hs-CRP blood test along with a cholesterol and blood pressure test and know their family history of heart disease, there is a new and wonderful risk assessment tool that I highly recommend, called the Reynolds Risk Score. Go to www.reynoldsriskscore.org to determine your risk. Print it out and take it to your doctor.

For Men Only
Calculate Your 10-Year Risk of Heart Disease for Men
(also called the Framingham risk score)

A. Find your age and point value and circle it.

Age (years)	Points
20–34	−9
35–39	−4
40–44	0
45–49	3
50–54	6
55–59	8
60–64	10
65–69	11
70–74	12
75–79	13

B. Find your total cholesterol level, match it to your age group, and then determine your point value and circle it.

Total Cholesterol (mg/dL or mmol/L)	Age 20–39	Age 40–49	Age 50–59	Age 60–69	Age 70–79
<160 or <4.14	0	0	0	0	0
160–199 or 4.15–5.16	4	3	2	1	0
200–239 or 5.18–6.19	7	5	3	1	0
240–279 or 6.22–7.23	9	6	4	2	1
≥280 or ≥7.25	11	8	5	3	1

C. If you are a current smoker or not, find your age group and find your point value and circle it.

Smoking Status Currently	Age 20–39	Age 40–49	Age 50–59	Age 60–69	Age 70–79
Nonsmoker	0	0	0	0	0
Smoker	8	5	3	1	1

D. Locate your HDL number and point value, and circle the point value.

HDL (mg/dL)	Points
≥60	−1
50–59	0
40–49	1
<40	2

E. Locate your systolic blood pressure, treated or untreated by medication, and find your point value and circle it.

Systolic BP (mmHg)	Untreated	Treated
<120	0	0
120–129	0	1
130–139	1	2
140–159	1	2
≥160	2	3

F. Add your circled points from A through E.

Age	Points =
Total cholesterol	Points =
Smoker/nonsmoker	Points =
HDL	Points =
Systolic blood pressure	Points =
Total points	_____

G. Match your total points from F to the table below, circle your 10-year risk of CHD, and bring it to your doctor on your next visit.

Total Points	10-Year Risk
<0	<1%
0–4	1%
5–6	2%
7	3%
8	4%
9	5%
10	6%
11	8%
12	10%
13	12%
14	16%
15	20%
16	25%
≥17	≥30%

Your Goal: Determine your 10-year Coronary Heart Disease (CHD) risk from the Framingham and Reynolds risk tests (www.reynoldsriskscore.org). Bring the results to your next doctor's visit.

Step 6 around the B.S.—Size and Shape

| Dr. B.S.

"If you want to lose weight, you first need to have your weight or BMI measured."

| Dr. Moyad's No B.S.

"Whatever! Forget about just losing weight; I really want you to eventually become fit and then lose some waist!"

Your weight (in pounds or kilograms) = _____
Your height (in inches or meters) = _____
Body mass index (BMI) = lbs/inches^2 × 704 or kg/m^2 = ____

Waist circumference (WC) or waist size = _____ (inches or cm)
Note: Your tape measure should be placed around the belly button area, but the official way to measure it is to find the halfway point between the bottom of the rib cage (costal margin) and the area of your hip that sticks out in front of your body (iliac crest).

Hip size = _____ (inches or cm)
Note: The hips for this purpose are the largest area around your buttocks.

Waist-to-hip ratio (WHR) = Waist size/hip measurement = _____

Current waist size of your pants = _____
(Note: Apart from all the official medical stuff, the current waist size of your pants is an easy way to see how you are doing.)

What Does the Body Mass Index (BMI) Number Mean?

BMI Number	What does this mean?
<25	Normal weight
25–29	Overweight
≥30	Obese

What Does the Waist Circumference (WC) Number Mean?

WC Number	What does this mean?
<35 inches (or <89 cm) in men	Normal
35–39 inches (or 89–100 cm) in men	Overweight
≥40 inches (≥101 cm) in men	Obese
<32.5 inches (or < 83 cm) in women	Normal
32.5–36 inches (or 83–92 cm) in women	Overweight
≥37 inches (≥94 cm) in women	Obese

What Does the Waist-to-Hip Ratio (WHR) Number Mean?

WHR Number	What does this mean?
<0.9	Low risk
0.9–1.0	Moderate risk
>1.0	High risk

B.S. Note: A new study says a WHR greater than 0.80 in women is unhealthy, and greater than 0.9 for men is unhealthy. All of these numbers are really B.S. because you are *competing against yourself* and not another person or some standard.

Dr. Moyad, what is the problem or catch with the BMI measurement and liposuction?

The real problem in humans is *visceral fat* (found deep around the liver, intestines, stomach ...) compared to *subcutaneous fat*, which is found right underneath your belly skin. Deep belly fat or visceral fat can cause problems, whereas subcutaneous fat is not necessarily unhealthy beyond being unsightly or unattractive to some people. This is also why, if you have a liposuction procedure that removes 10 or 20 pounds of subcutaneous fat, you may look better, but your cholesterol level and blood pressure will usually not decrease. However, if you lose an inch or more of visceral fat or deep belly fat, your cholesterol and blood pressure will generally drop almost immediately!

BMI does not take into account where your weight is distributed (on the waist or on the hips). If you lift weights, as all of us should, it can increase your BMI because you are increasing lean muscle mass. The increased BMI is going to imply that you are getting fatter, when in fact you are becoming healthier and more toned! So, this is why the waist size of your pants, WC, and WHR are more important numbers.

Your Goal: Weigh yourself and measure your height and waist and hip size. All of these measurements will allow you to calculate your body mass index (BMI), waist circumference, waist-to-hip ratio (WHR), or, being newly used, your waist-to-height ratio, to give you a better idea of your risk. Lower numbers are better.

Step 7 around the B.S.—Family Health Tree

| Dr. B.S.

"Genetic tests that better personalize medicine are very promising and will be the wave of the future (circa 1985)!"

| Dr. Moyad's No B.S.

"It is a slow process to develop genetic tests, and there are already other traditional, less-expensive tests available to determine your risk of various diseases. So, sit down with the family, including the kids, and go over your family health history tree, and not only you but also your children will learn from it the importance of basic prevention."

Family Health History Review

Family Member	Overall Health & Age (Include diagnosis of condition/disease and age at diagnosis)	Status (Living/deceased; if deceased include cause of death and age at death)
Grandfather (paternal)		
Grandfather (maternal)		
Grandmother (paternal)		
Grandmother (maternal)		
Father		

Family Member	Overall Health & Age (Include diagnosis of condition/disease and age at diagnosis)	Status (Living/deceased; if deceased include cause of death and age at death)
Mother		
Brother(s)		
Sister(s)		
Other Family Members (uncles, aunts, cousins)		

Your Goal: Fill out your entire family health or disease tree so that you and your doctor can understand any family history of possible disease risks.

Step 8 around the B.S.—Screening Tests

| Dr. B.S.

"Early detection is the key to preventive medicine because if you find it early you still have a chance to cure it."

| Dr. Moyad's No B.S.

"Whatever! Early detection seems logical, but if there is no evidence to support it or the risk-to-benefit ratio is not completely explained, it can be illogical. If consumers working with their doctors prioritize some early detection test(s) based on probability of what may or may not end their lives early or their quality of life early, compared to later or never ... well, now you have something that may be beneficial versus something potentially harmful."

In addition to the list below, go to www.ahrq.gov for a complete list of tests endorsed by the U.S. Preventive Services Task Force. Some of these tests can be expensive—inquire as to cost and insurance coverage.

Screening Test	Dr. Moyad's Comments
Bone Health Screening	
DEXA	DEXA or dual energy X-ray absorptiometry measures bone mineral density. This test is safe, effective, and the gold standard test for osteoporosis. A few people will need a quantitative CT scan.
FRAX	The World Health Organization's tool to assess the 10-year probability of bone fracture can be accessed and used at www.shef.ac.uk./FRAX/
Breast Cancer/Health Screening	
Breast Self/Clinical Exam	Early detection can reduce the risk of dying from this disease. Do it!
Mammography	Recommendations for age at initial mammogram and frequency of test vary.

Screening Test	Dr. Moyad's Comments
MRI test and/or Genetic BRCA1/2	For high-risk individuals including those with multiple relatives with breast cancer at an early age (premenopausal), bilateral breast tumors, a family history of breast and/or ovarian cancer, dense breast tissue, or breast cancer in one or more male family members
Cardiovascular Health Screening	
Ultrasonography for Abdominal Aortic Aneurysm (AAA)	One-time AAA screening is approved and recommended for men 65 years and over who do smoke or have smoked.
Ankle-Brachial Index (ABI)	ABI is a simple way to screen for peripheral artery disease by comparing blood pressure between the upper and lower body.
Carotid duplex ultrasound (CDUS) and a stethoscope option	CDUS is a simple way to screen for those at a high risk of a stroke. The procedure uses ultrasound to look for plaques, blood clots, or other blood flow problems in the carotid arteries. The carotid arteries, located in the neck, supply blood to the brain.
Executive physical	Executive physicals with comprehensive tests and lengthy doctor consultations review your cardiac health from head to toe!
MRI screening of the head for risk of brain aneurysm	Recommended only for those with a strong family history (like Dr. Moyad)
Cervical Cancer/Health Screening	
Pap Smear (& Additional Methods)	Proven to reduce deaths, period! (Ask your doctor)
HPV Vaccine	HPV vaccine and side effects should be explained to and discussed with every young woman.
Colon Cancer/Health Screening	
Colonoscopy	Should be mandatory at the age of 50 for women and men, but especially women because they tend to get polyps higher up in the colon. You can be awake or not during this *(continued)*

	test, so talk to the doctor about which option is best for you. "Virtual" colonoscopy is a new and expensive test with high radiation exposure. If abnormalities are found during the test, you then have the standard colonoscopy. So just cut to the chase and get the real thing.
Dental Health Screening	Ask your dentist or doctor about oral cancer screening. During a routine checkup, they will look for lesions in your mouth. Taking care of your teeth translates into better overall health.
Eye Health Screening	
Glaucoma Test	The purpose of this test (and there are variations) is to measure the pressure inside your eye.
Complete Eye Examination	A whole range of eye conditions and diseases can be detected with a complete eye exam, including cataracts, macular degeneration, corneal ulcers, and diabetic eye disease.
Amsler Grid (for macular degeneration)	To monitor vision between eye exams, self-testing can be done online at www.eyesight.org.
Hearing Health Screening	Simple and easy to do. Not usually done in adults, which is a shame.
Lung/Respiratory Health Screening	Procedure can range from the doctor listening to your lungs with a stethoscope to a chest X-ray to a discussion of allergies and any other breathing issues, such as those that occur during sleep.
Mental/Brain Health Screening (including depression, stress, energy levels, memory testing, blood tests)	Discuss depression, stress, energy levels, and memory testing with your doctor. If you have a high risk for Alzheimer's, ask your doctor about an Apo E blood screening test.
Ovarian/Testicular/ Reproductive Cancer Screening	The blood test (CA-125) is not an effective screening test for ovarian cancer. *(continued)*

Screening Test	Dr. Moyad's Comments
	Discussing these subjects relies on very good communication between doctor and patient in terms of past and recent symptoms.
Prostate Cancer Screening	
Digital Rectal Exam (DRE)	Simple and inexpensive
Prostate-Specific Antigen (PSA)	Best possible blood test after being treated for prostate cancer. Non-cancerous prostate enlargement increases PSA more than a cancer, and infections of the prostate also increase PSA.
Sexual Health Screening Includes erectile function, female sexual function, sexual desire or libido, and male and female hormone levels.	Discussing these subjects relies on very good communication between doctor and patient.
Skin Cancer Screening	Educate yourself about sunscreen. Skin cancer kills quickly, so anyone at high risk should consider mole mapping (full-body photography to track changes in existing or the development of new moles). Only suspicious or high-risk moles should be removed.
Sleep Pattern Screening	Includes a simple discussion of sleep patterns to possibly more clinical testing/ polysomnography for real sleep problems. The health impacts of sleep deprivation are getting more attention, because it may increase the risk of a variety of diseases.
Thyroid Disease/Health Screening	Simple blood testing of your thyroid levels or possibly an imaging test.
Vaccines Up-to-Date Review	Vaccines can improve your chances of living longer. Remember the rotavirus oral vaccine for babies, cervical cancer vaccine for young women, meningitis vaccine for high school and college students, shingles and pneumococcal vaccines for older individuals, and seasonal flu vaccine for almost everyone.

Dr. Moyad, should I have a full body screen or scan?

Next time you want a full body screen, remember that you are getting the equivalent of about 100 to 200 X-rays (depending on the device) every time you get one test! (Look Mom, I glow in the dark!)

Your Goal: Discuss screening tests with your doctor to see which ones you need and which ones you should avoid for now and in the future.

Step 9 around the B.S.—Health in the Workplace

Congratulations. After this section you will have cleared the first large pile of Bogus Science. This is possibly the most critical step.

Let's put your risk assessment all together in one piece and move forward, but realize that this cannot take place unless you have seriously considered workplace health.

| Dr. B.S.

"If you want to become healthier just follow this simple tip ... blah, blah, blah ... that I put in a paper or a magazine and just listen to me blah, blah, blah ... it is that easy."

| Dr. Moyad's No B.S.

"Whatever! This is one of the more embarrassing parts about reading quickie types of health advice from B.S. experts ... the notion that you just need to follow a few simple steps because your life is supposed to mirror theirs. This is absurd! The best advice I can give you is that you need to ask yourself two questions: (1) Does your work/life schedule revolve around your health or vice versa? (2) Can you go out and find health where you or your doctor never knew it existed?"

Here comes another Moyad personal story (sorry, folks).

I used to schedule my travel around my work or lectures, so I would fly in and fly out (red-eye or not), and I thought I was the man when really I was an idiot! I used to commute to school or the hospital, balancing two full-time jobs, and I thought I was the man, but I was, again, a big idiot. I would counsel all types of individuals who were as reckless as I was until, over a very long period of time, I realized I needed to stop listening to the B.S.! The question this brings up is how can you improve the entire health of a nation without some national health care plan? How can you improve the health of our kids without bringing back recess or physical education or health class five days a week? How can you improve the health of our adult nation without allowing the employee time to become healthier at work? In other words, *unless we eventually allow our schedules or life to revolve around our health* and not vice versa, it is difficult to achieve or experience our true mental and physical health capacity.

So our family moved to a smaller house near the hospital, and we now use one car. I generally walk to work; my wife and son walk or bike to school. In the past two years, this has allowed our family to reach what I finally believe is our maximum physical and mental health. I deal with patients now who have put exercise equipment in the workplace or make sure, before flying to a meeting, that the hotel has a 24-hour workout center. I try to show patients that when they spend several hundred dollars on the latest and greatest supreme form of health food or expensive supplements that there is a less obvious price to pay! So, they start paying less and using the money on more healthy things such as that occasional trip to paradise or that piece of health equipment, dance or spinning class ... whatever ... but at least their lives become more balanced.

The greater point here is how can we become more healthy unless the rest of our lives revolves around our health, and the answer lies in the place we are required to spend most of our time. Most of us need to get more time to work on our health *at work*! Everyone eventually wins here, because the employer pays less in health-care costs and productivity and loyalty increase, while the employee becomes healthier, including mentally, which means her or his private life should also improve. The task is difficult here but worth it ... ask your employer for some exercise time several days at work, or begin to organize a group that can eventually open up an exercise facility or room at your workplace; or, if there is an exercise facility near work, see if your company can work out a deal whereby the employees can become healthier by using this facility.

It is interesting that when you talk to doctors or other health-care workers over the years at many of the most prestigious centers, they often say how much easier it was to get a patient to quit smoking when the patient's employer did not allow smoking in the workplace or provided some support for quitting. In other words, they felt more effective when the workplace provided some support around their advice. This concept of exercise in the workplace also works by positive reinforcement!

Finally, it is easy for me to also mention the obvious, such as do not smoke, exercise regularly, eat right, get sleep ... blah, blah, blah. Anyone can do that, but finding health where you did not know it existed should be attempted on a regular basis—or, I like to say, at least once a year! So for me, living near work was the smartest thing I did, or stopping the red-eye flights, or cooking with my wife or … so ask yourself if you can find health where you didn't know it existed, and surprise yourself and your doctor!

So, now let me ask you again. Does your life/work revolve around your health or does your health revolve around your life/work?

Oh, and for those that have already made up their minds that their employer or boss would never allow exercise of any kind during the work week … well, I have provided you with a doctor's note below.

Dear Mrs./Ms./Mr./Boss

My name is Dr. Mark A. Moyad, and I work in the area of Preventive Medicine at the University of Michigan Medical Center. I am one of the only doctors around the world who get to work and teach other doctors/health-care professionals full time (not part time) about how to make their patients healthier by using preventive medicine such as lifestyle changes in their daily lives. So, now your employee _____ read my book, and I have instructed this person that the smartest thing they can do for their health is start getting some exercise time during the workday in order to *reduce employer health-care costs and improve company loyalty and productivity*. I am asking you to work with this obviously motivated person to allow them several hours a week in a variety of capacities that they or I can explain to improve their health in order to ultimately improve the financial health of your company/business.

I really appreciate your time. All the best,

Mark A. Moyad, MD, MPH

Your Goal: Find new opportunities to improve your mental and physical health.

Step 10—More Than the Physical

Before you delve into more information about cholesterol and blood tests, your disease risk factors, or physical screening tests, I would like to share some other "heart" information. Whether emotions come from our hearts or some part of our brains, they do affect our physical well-being. The minister of my church and my wife have shared stories with me, and I would like to include them here.

Spirituality

Spirituality begins with the recognition of our intrinsic value as human beings, an appreciation for the inner workings of self-consciousness, and an acknowledgment of our connectedness with others and with all of life. To be a spiritual person then means to live with a deeper awareness of life and self, along with the life forces that surround us day by day.

Practically speaking, our overall health and wellness are affected and often improved as we attend to the nurture of our spiritual side. Here, such things as seeking the best for self and others, expecting good outcomes, living with hope and gratitude, believing in a benevolent God or universe, imaging healing and light, accepting mystery, finding new pathways for solving problems, pursuing inner peace, living with optimism, thinking positively, creating harmony in one's relationships, as well as other factors influence how we feel and impact our general state of well-being.

Let me share a story with you. One summer I took a group of high school youth and adults to the Boundary Waters Wilderness Canoe Area in northern Minnesota for a week of canoeing and camping. On our second day out, we needed to cross a huge lake to get to the portage point to another lake where we would be camping that night. Vested with map and compass, one of our youth volunteered to be our navigator for the day. So off we went! It was tough canoeing that day because of stiff winds and choppy waters, but nonetheless we plodded forward. However, after a few of hours of paddling, one of the other campers wondered why we hadn't come to our portage point yet. We decided to stop and take a look at the map. To our chagrin and to the horror of our young navigator, we found that we had been paddling in the wrong direction for most of the day, and we now had an even longer way to go to get to where we needed to be. To say the least, our group was feeling both annoyed and dismayed. After all, our group was getting tired, and the thought of having to go farther than expected created a good deal of tension. Offering up a silent prayer, I asked if anyone had any thoughts or ideas to share with the group before we returned to our canoes and headed on our way. First, one camper spoke up and wanted to offer forgiveness and encouragement to our navigator, saying that anyone could have made the same mistake. Then another camper talked about what a beautiful day it was, and how lucky we were to be up in the wilderness. Finally a third camper addressed the group and suggested that, since the wind would now be at our backs, perhaps if we took the eight-by-ten camping tarp out of our tent pack, tied our four canoes together side-by-side, and used the tarp and our canoe paddles to make a makeshift sail, we could sail across the lake. Though some scoffed at the idea, we decided to give it a try, and it worked! What started out as a defeat and a downer turned out to be an afternoon of fun, laughter, community, healing, wholeness, and personal triumph.

Such is the power and essence of spirituality, and such is its potential impact on our health and sense of wellness. As Winston Churchill once quipped, "You create your own universe as you go along." A positive, uplifting spirituality helps.

—Robert K. Livingston
Senior Minister
The First Congregational Church of Ann Arbor, Michigan

The Importance of Helping

(This example comes from my wonderful partner, best friend, and wife, who wrote this piece in our local paper ... it really says it all.)

"On October 21, I lost my beautiful, wonderful, full-of-life sister, Tawn Mastrey, to a deficient liver. She was one of the most important people in the world to me. She died from complications of hepatitis C. If you are already an organ donor, I thank you and your potential recipient thanks you! If you are not yet on the national registry, please read on. Our nation is suffering from a silent epidemic known as hepatitis C. It is considered an epidemic because the number of infected people has increased by 49 percent in the past 10 years.

Approximately 4 million people are infected with the virus; this is almost 2 percent of the population. This is four times greater than the population of those infected with HIV/AIDS. This illness also carries a stigma similar to HIV/AIDS due to transmission similarities, and there seems to be the same reluctance to talk about it, and support it. We are currently losing approximately 10,000 people a year, but this number is expected to climb in the next 3 to 10 years. We will be spending an estimated $85 billion between the years 2010 and 2019. While we have had a 67 percent increase in organ donors in the past decade, we have also had a 49 percent increase in organs needed, so we are still not meeting the demand. As of today we have 97,934 people waiting for the call to say, "Yes, we have an organ for you!" Seventeen of those people will die today. Statistics show that face-to-face conversation is the best way to educate people about this need, to encourage them to register to be a donor. If I could, I would meet with each one of you reading this today to implore you to please register yourself on the donor list. Unfortunately, I cannot. However, I can make the process extremely easy for you. If you have a computer just go online to register at www.organdonor.org/register.html.

—Mia M. Moyad
(Friday, December 14, 2007,
on page A10 in the *Ann Arbor News*)

Your Goal: When having all the other tests listed in this book, don't forget to self-administer a "spirituality screening." Have you donated blood, added your name to the bone marrow registry, taken a CPR educational class, or signed up for organ donation? All of these rely on volunteering or educating yourself to help others, realizing that your good health is a gift that does others no good unless it is shared.

To contact the National Bone Marrow Donor Program and sign up as a bone marrow or cord blood donor to help save lives: www.marrow.org

To contact the National Transplant Society and sign up to be an organ donor to help save lives: www.organdonor.org

To contact the American Red Cross on how to learn CPR, or how to use an automated external defibrillator (AED) device, or how to give first aid or how to give blood to help save lives: www.redcross.org and www.givelife.org (for where to go locally to donate blood).

To donate to the Lower Ninth Ward Free Health Clinic in New Orleans (5228 St. Claude Avenue, New Orleans, LA 70117) or another important health charity that is near and dear to your heart, please check the web for the latest phone numbers and web sites.

Review

You should know your exact cardiovascular disease (CVD) risk by now, so if I ask you the numbers you need to know from Part I, you can repeat them to me as quickly as you could repeat your birth date and your anniversary or even the teacher or the boy/girl you disliked and liked the most in high school! Let's do a basic review.

What is your total cholesterol? _____

What is your goal for your next total cholesterol test? _____

What is your LDL? _____

What is your goal for your next LDL test? _____

What is your HDL? _____

What is your goal for your next HDL test? _____

What is your triglyceride number? _____

What is your goal for your next triglyceride test? _____

What is your hs-CRP or other blood tests? _____

What is your goal for your next hs-CRP test? _____

Have you purchased a blood pressure monitoring kit? _____

What is your blood pressure? _____

What is your goal in the next year for your blood pressure? _____

What is your Framingham Risk Score? _____

How can you reduce your Framingham Risk Score?
_____

For *women only*, what is your Reynolds Risk Score? _____

How can you reduce your Reynolds Risk Score?
_____

What is your waist circumference (WC) and waist-hip ratio (WHR)? _____

Where would you like your WC and WHR to be in the next year?
_____

What is the waist size of your pants, what would you like it to be in the next year? _____ and _____.

What does your family health history look like, and what is your biggest worry after looking over your family disease/health tree?

(Note: You cannot answer this question by saying that your biggest worry is that your husband or wife will look like his father or her mother one day even though many of us are completely and legitimately concerned about this issue ... not me ... I mean some of my friends.)

What are you considering for your spiritual health project?

(Note: Never answer, "Well, I just want to help people," "help children," or "be a good dad or mom or friend" ... blah, blah, blah, *because you are supposed to do that anyway!*)

What is the result of your 25-OH vitamin D test? _____

What number do you want it to be on your next vitamin D test? _____

Part II

Dr. Moyad's No B.S.
Dietary & Lifestyle Changes

(Should have named this part "How *Not* to Have a Ridiculous &
Unhealthy Obsession with Health That Many B.S. Experts Support,"
or should have named this part "The Mostly Pill-Free Zone!")

**Please remember: Heart Healthy = All Healthy
and Heart Unhealthy = All Unhealthy!**

Basic education is the best diet. Life is too short to follow one person's specific ideas from the cradle to the grave, so most of the lifestyle and dietary recommendations in this section are just general rules to follow!

Remember, you should first reduce your *cardiovascular* risk to as close to *zero* as possible, because this is a high-probability event that *we know* you can reduce!

Have you completed part I and the review questions? If yes, go to step 11; and if not, come on and get off your small, medium, or big gluteus maximus and go back and finish part I.

Step 11 in the B.S.—Dr. Moyad's Favorite Pill

Take this pill first before you do anything else in this book.

Okay, so below I will first present the results of this cheap pill and why I recommend it to almost everyone, including all health-care professionals. But please, only try and take it once per day. The price of this pill can vary, so do not pay too much for it!

| Dr. B.S.

"Let me tell you about the latest and greatest supplement or drug!"

| Dr. Moyad's No B.S.

"Whatever! I tell you what, I will tell you about the latest and greatest supplement or drug after you first tell me specifically what your latest heart disease risk numbers are and what your numbers should be at this point in your life for optimum health. What the heck, let me tell you about the greatest dietary supplement or pill first, and perhaps then we can talk about dietary changes!"

Note: Step 11 is against everything I believe, but I am going to talk to you about my *favorite pill in the world*.

Here are the results from a systematic review of the literature from the largest human studies on the latest pill that you should take almost every day. (Research shows that if you do not take this pill regularly, the benefits quickly go away!)

Health Condition	Reduction in Risk when a Woman or Man, Regardless of Age, Takes This Preventive Pill
Alzheimer's disease & some other types of dementia	30–40%
Breast cancer	20–30%
Colon cancer	30–50%
Depression	25–50%
Erectile dysfunction (ED)	25–50%
Female sexual dysfunction (FSD)	25–50%
Heart disease (& all types of CVD)	40–50%
Osteoporosis	40–50%
Parkinson's disease	Unknown percentage, but this pill at least reduces the risk (recent finding)
Premature death (sudden death)	30–50%
Prostate cancer, prostatitis, prostate enlargement	25–50%
Stroke	30–50%
Type II diabetes	30–40%
Dying early after being diagnosed/treated for most of the above diseases	Reduced also (studies even suggest less aggressive forms of these diseases are more likely in people who take this cheap pill)

So, the pill that is without question associated with all these risk reductions is ...

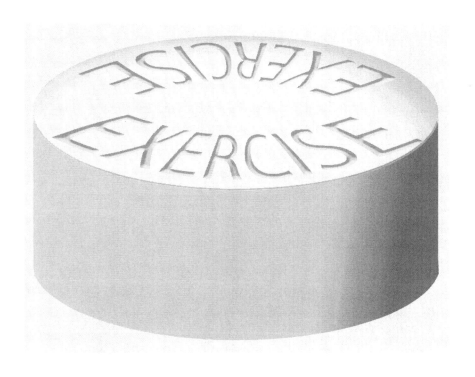

Did you notice how step 11 said "in the B.S." and not "around the B.S."? Did you pick up on that? Well I did that because I just B.S.ed you! Sorry, but I could not resist. And this is why you were B.S.ed.—because if I had introduced this as exercise, half of you would have skipped this part. *The good news is that in research it really did not matter what kind of exercise you did just as long as you were getting about 30 minutes a day average.* Pills are great, but first understand the power of one of the greatest "pills" ever invented. If you truly understand and believe that power, it makes it that much easier to exercise!

If you need even more motivation to take the pill on the previous page, just look at the disease risk reduction that occurs with regular use. Tear the table out of the book and carry it with you to the gym. If you pretend that the numbers in the table are what you get with a supplement or a prescription drug, you know you would be taking that pill every day.

The only reason I try to (note the words "try to") exercise four to seven days a week, every week, regardless of where I am in the world, is that I wrote the table above and memorized it over the years. It just kept growing to the point where I knew damn well that if those numbers represented a pill (supplement or drug), I would take it almost every single day for the rest of my life. I am not going to B.S. you; I do not exercise daily because I always love it or just feel like I have to look healthy for a talk. I exercise now to maintain and improve my health.

Please do not give me an Uncle Fred or Aunt Mary story, which is where you tell me that you had this person in your family or someone you knew who exercised all the time and never ate anything bad and died young of a heart attack, while another uncle/aunt/friend never did anything healthy and lived to be 101 years old, and then you ask me to explain it. Life is a probability game. I will take my chances on learning from the thousands of normal examples rather than the one or two abnormal examples, even though it provides no guarantee for a longer and better life—just a higher probability or chance of one. This is the same philosophy that has me wearing a seat belt or buying a smoke detector or carbon monoxide detector for my home. (Every home should have a carbon monoxide detector!)

The Real Step 11 around the B.S.

"Everything in life comes with a catch or a risk-to-benefit ratio, and I mean everything! So, you have to decide if it is worth it. If I ask you to go running a few days a week, you are going to get healthier but a few of you out of a million will either twist an ankle, get a piece of your butt chomped on by a vicious dog, or maybe even get hit by a bus!"

—Dr. Moyad, circa now

| Dr. B.S.

"Specific exercises are better than others, and the best time to exercise is in the morning, so you are done for the day. Also, only use certain types of muscles on one day and other types on another day, and free weights are better than other types of resistance machines."

| Dr. Moyad's No B.S.

"Whatever! All types of exercise or physical activity are just fine, and it really does not matter when or where you exercise as long as you just do it. Finally, it does not matter what type of weight-lifting program or equipment is recommended to you, because you should do the type of weight lifting (like your aerobic exercise) that keeps you interested in doing this healthy thing for the rest of your life!"

Exercise comes in a variety of forms, and you should pick the one that works for you long term. Some people like to walk or walk stairs, others like to swim or row or use a treadmill or use an elliptical machine—there are many activities from which to choose. Some people with joint pain or other pain issues can work out in a swimming pool. The amount of physical activity you do and how frequently you do it are dependent on your weight. An individual should do, at the least, enough exercise to help him or her maintain a healthy weight. Some patients have to exercise every day for 30 minutes, while others only have to exercise 3 or 4 days a week. Obviously, the more active you are the better. Personally, I like to exercise for 30 to 45 minutes a day for about 5 days a week. After a few months I get sick of this routine, and I will just do one hour of exercise every other day to give my brain, joints, and delicate Joe Namath–like knees a rest.

An additional benefit noted in recent research is that exercise promotes good *mental health*, because it seems to reduce the risk of depression or recurrence after depression.

If you are interested, the following table is for Exercise Zone Training for a variety of workouts—elliptical, stationary bike, treadmill …

Age	Minimal Exercise Heart Rate* (65% effort = low intensity = fat-burning time)	Maximum Exercise Heart Rate* (80% effort = high intensity = heart-healthy time)
10	136	168
20	130	160
30	123	152
40	117	144
50	110	136
60	104	128
70	97	120
80	91	112
90	84	104
100	78	96
110	Who cares? You should not be reading my book; I should be reading yours!	Who cares? You should not be reading my book; I should be reading yours!

*Note: This is the suggested target heart rate as a percentage of your maximum heart rate range, which is 55–90 percent, according to many established organizations or groups.

Dr. Moyad, what is more important in general, exercise four to five times a week or run a marathon once a week?

It is better to exercise frequently because the human body seems to respond *mentally and physically* as it would to a cholesterol-lowering or other type of drug or effective pill. In other words, if you look at your HDL or "good cholesterol," frequency of exercise really impacts you more and not the duration of exercise. Clearly this is how the mental health benefits of exercise work. Give me a patient who walks or runs four to five days a week for 30 minutes, and I will show you a much happier and healthy person compared to the crabby-pants guy or gal who only runs a long distance one day a week!

Another important tip for those of you who thought your body does not respond to abuse ... it does, in my opinion, in the form of early death! I am dumbfounded traveling the world at times and watching health-care professionals, or anyone for that matter, exercising *without much sleep, or ill, or in really high or low temperatures.* When did these people decide that they were as tough as the military boot camp dudes and dudettes? The human body is like a car—if you run it constantly without rest and without oil changes and tune-ups, there is a good chance it will break down on you. If you run it through Death Valley often enough when it is 125 degrees outside, there is a good chance it can break down. If you try and start it and run it often enough in Anchorage, Alaska, at 30 degrees below freezing, there is a good chance it will not last long. When did we decide we were exempt from this rule? Sudden cardiac death among exercisers is uncommon, but common enough that it is still a problem. My personal research suggests it is more common in individuals who really exercised with great intensity when the body was not able to handle this stress. I tell patients not to exercise or lift weights when they are sick, have not slept, are in an unhealthy environment like extremely high or low temperatures, or just off a 100-hour work week. It is no B.S. to start realizing that being unhealthy or being in an unhealthy place or environment is *never* the time to think you are ready for exercise!

Dr. Moyad, I see this thing on exercise equipment known as "mets," so what the heck is that?

It is important to understand the definition of a metabolic equivalent task (MET) score. A single MET is the energy that is expended by just sitting quietly. MET scores are used by some researchers to calculate the average intensity of a specific exercise. MET scores for specific exercises are defined as the ratio of the metabolic rate associated with a specific activity divided by the resting metabolic rate. For example, if someone walks at an average pace the person is generally assigned a MET score of 3; jogging, a MET score of 7; and running, a MET score of 12. The higher the number of METs during your exercise routine, the greater the workout for your heart. You will see this the next time you get on an exercise machine that reports METs.

Weight lifting is probably as important as aerobic or regular exercise.

Weight Lifting Benefits

Medical Area	Do we see an improvement from weight lifting just 2 to 3 times a week?
Bone health	Yes! Stimulates bone growth and reduces the risk of osteoporosis, and improves strength, balance, and coordination to reduce the risk of falls and bone fracture.
Cardiovascular health	Yes! Exercises the heart muscle (Note: If you have a heart condition like an aortic aneurysm or dissection, many doctors do not want you to lift weights ... I agree.)
Energy levels/Mood/ Fatigue	Yes! Reduces fatigue by as much as 50% in some studies. Improves energy levels by increasing the efficiency of the body to produce energy. All of this means an increased chance of improved mood during the entire day!
Joint health	Yes! Lifting weights and strength training cause muscles to grow and become stronger, reducing the amount of weight or pressure on the joint, and may improve or prevent osteoarthritic problems.
Muscle health	Yes! We all know this, but by increasing lean muscle mass it helps not only to improve overall strength but also to make you burn calories more effectively.
Neurologic health	Yes! Improves balance and increases insulin sensitivity of the body so it lowers blood glucose and allows the electrical wiring of the body to work more effectively.
Blood sugar health/ Diabetes	Yes! Improves the body's ability to maintain a normal sugar level by increasing the sensitivity of your cells to insulin, so it can reduce your risk of diabetes or improve your diabetes!
Waist & weight loss	Yes! Yes! Yes! Perhaps the most effective way to lose waist & weight, because more lean muscle mass means a faster metabolism and improved body appearance or tone!

Dr. Moyad, are you a bonehead? Every doctor says lift weights, but what kind of weights (free weights, Nautilus® ...) and for how long?

Don't get personal here and do not get obsessed here. The simplest set of weight-lifting exercises is enough to improve your health. If you do not believe me that simplicity is the answer, well ... let me show you one of the largest randomized clinical trials of weight lifting to improve health and energy, and let me show the actual weight-lifting exercise these participants did 2–3 times a week for 30 minutes. By the way, there are enough studies to suggest that free weights or Nautilus-type weights are just fine.

Weight-Lifting Exercise (Just a suggestion, not an obsession. Please do not make loud grunting noises when you lift weights in a public gym.)	Initial Repetition (The lowest weight with which you are comfortable. Please do not try to emulate Schwarzenegger or Jack LaLanne at the beginning.)	Additional Repetition (plus 2.5–5 lbs. or 1–2 kg of weight)
Biceps curl	12 to 15	8 to 10
Chest press	12 to 15	8 to 10
Latissimus pull-down	12 to 15	8 to 10
Modified curl-ups	12 to 15	8 to 10
Overhead press	12 to 15	8 to 10
Triceps extension	12 to 15	8 to 10
Calf raises	12 to 15	8 to 10
Leg curl	12 to 15	8 to 10
Leg extension	12 to 15	8 to 10
Moyad spine bone building exercise*	8 to 12 modified push-ups	8 to 12 modified push-ups

*Some doctors or trainers like to include a back lift in order to strengthen the spine. A small or low weight that is shaped like a small sac, cushion, bag, or pillow (just a few pounds or kilograms) is placed on the upper back between the shoulder blades. While lying on your stomach, you do 8–12 modified push-ups (stomach stays on the pillow, hands clasped together on the back of your head, and lift your upper body up then down, up and down). This places resistance on the spine and may improve bone mineral density in this area.

Get your doctor's approval before starting any resistance or weight-bearing program!

Dr. Moyad says remember to:

- Talk to your employer about how to get more exercise time in your workday.
- Pick exercise(s) that you enjoy. Getting some activity every day is critical to maintain or improve your mental health. Begin to give weight lifting the same importance as aerobic exercise.
- Eventually throw the pedometer out (that's right, I said it) and begin to learn how much exercise you need on your own. I can just about guarantee that if you buy a pedometer, within the first year it will generally end up in the same closet with the Vibrating Abdominal Fat Shrinking Machine and all those other things that don't work and you don't need.
- Buy a durable and fun piece of exercise equipment before you buy a new car. This and other behaviors send a clear message that compared to everything else your health has to come first!
- Swimming, of course, counts as exercise, and even doing water exercises is a good way for people who need to do a low-impact exercise because of knee problems, arthritis, and other conditions. It burns calories effectively, but the biggest concern with swimming or water exercise is the lack of benefit to bone health. Resistance exercise (or weight lifting) needs to be done to get these benefits.
- Keep in mind that the largest human clinical studies in the world have clearly shown that if two people are equal in weight, and one person exercises regularly compared to the other person, the person who exercises regularly has a far greater chance of living longer and better. This is why weight loss should not be the initial concern, but rather just fitness!

B.S. Cathartic/Cleansing Moment!

Finally, three more B.S. things that need to be discussed right now.

- Stretching is overrated! That's right, I said it! It is better to warm up the muscles by walking for 5 to 10 minutes than to try to contort and hurt yourself. Yeah, I fell for this B.S., too.

I used to stretch before running as much as the 1972 Soviet gymnastics team, because I was told how it prevents injury! However, there were no basic studies. What seemed so logical turned out to cause more harm than good for some people. Stretching loosened up people too much, so it was easy to suffer a serious injury. By warming up through movement (like walking), it gives your muscles and joints an opportunity to gradually get used to the strenuous stuff.

- Sodium and simple sugar replacement is just as important as fluid replacement, especially after strenuous exercise! Look to find sports drinks that have more sodium in them, because researchers have realized that low sodium levels after strenuous exercise can be deadly. The body and brain need a certain level of sodium and simple sugar to function, and just drinking water can dilute your blood sodium level. Use some cheap candy chews during or after your workout.

- Caffeine is underrated! A few sips of a diet caffeinated soda or another small source of caffeine right before the workout or at halftime (during a break) is a legal way to enhance your exercise performance. Small amounts of caffeine can give you a better workout and may even reduce muscle fatigue.

Your Goal: Exercise or just move more, and this includes weight-lifting or resistance exercise. Do an *average* of 30 minutes a day or more of physical activity and lifting weights/resistance exercise at least two to three times a week. *Remember, fitness is initially much more important than weight loss.*

Step 12 around the B.S.—Maintain a Healthy Weight

Note: Step 12 is not a B.S. free zone. This is the one place in the book you may want to take advantage of the power of B.S. to help maintain a healthy weight.

| Dr. B.S.

"It is okay to be moderately overweight or obese as you get older!"

| Dr. Moyad's No B.S.

"Whatever! When was the last time you saw a moderately heavy-looking 90-year-old man or woman walking on the streets of China, Japan, anywhere else in Asia, the United States, or even in Europe? It is okay to be who you are, but let's not kid ourselves."

Dr. Moyad, what the heck is a calorie?

A calorie is the amount of heat or energy needed to raise the temperature of 1 gram or 1 kilogram of water 1 degree Celsius (this is equal to 4.184 Joules or 4.184 KJ). Whatever! So, if a food or beverage has 20 calories that means when it was burned it raised the temperature of the surrounding water by 20 degrees Celsius! Okay, now that I have wasted 20 seconds of your life let's get back to the important stuff.

Remember that 3,500 calories = approximately 1 pound (0.5 kilograms) of weight. This is very intimidating in terms of weight loss. However, if we rearrange this equation, the so-called glass really looks half-full and not half-empty. If you can cut back just 100 calories a day (418 kJ), which is the same amount as half a candy bar, we are talking of losing about 10 pounds (about 5 kilograms) in a year. Not bad! And, if you are able to cut back 200 calories a day, which is about the size of a candy bar, we are talking of losing about 20 pounds (about 10 kilograms) in a year! That is awesome! And oops!! I apologize for just revealing the secret of almost every fad diet ever invented! They all mostly operate on having you cut back about 100 to 200 calories a day, regardless of whether you notice it or not. For example, low-carb diets allow you to eat more fat or protein, which makes you feel more full, and you actually think you are eating more but you are actually eating less! How much less? About 100 to 200 calories a day.

So, you want to lose a ton (more or less) of weight? Why? Let's look at simple or small amounts of weight loss and what can be expected.

What Just 10% Weight Loss Can Do in Terms of Health Improvements
(for example, someone 250 pounds going to 225 pounds)

Medical Condition	Improvement in Health Numbers
Blood pressure	Reduction of about 10 mmHg in systolic and diastolic blood pressure in individuals with hypertension.
Cholesterol	Reduction of 10% in total cholesterol Reduction of 15% in LDL ("bad") cholesterol Increase of about 10% in HDL ("good") cholesterol Reduction of 30% in triglycerides
Diabetes	Reduction of as much as 50% in a fasting sugar (glucose) level of a newly diagnosed diabetic Reduction of about 30% in fasting insulin levels 30% increase in insulin sensitivity 40–60% reduction in the risk of getting diabetes
Mortality/Death	Reduction of at least 20% in risk of dying young from any cause Reduction of at least 30% in risk of death associated with diabetes Reduction of at least 40% in risks of death associated with obesity

Fat in your buttocks, legs, arms, or back is not the concern. Fat in the belly is the biggest concern because this can change hormone levels, cholesterol levels, and other levels in an unfavorable way. In fact, belly fat has been linked with a number of unhealthy changes listed here.

- Increases levels of estrogen and reduces testosterone in men. In women it increases estrogen and testosterone. In both genders, it simply causes unhealthy levels of male and female hormones.

- Increases the concentration of growth factors in fat tissue, which can be released into the body and stimulates the growth of unhealthy cells.
- Increases sugar and insulin levels.
- Increases nerve sympathetic activity, which can increase blood pressure and abnormally impact communication among cells of the body.
- Increases cholesterol levels that are unhealthy, especially tri-glycerides, and reduces levels of good cholesterol (HDL). Belly fat is actually stored as triglycerides.
- Causes abnormal immune system functioning and reduces immune defenses.
- Reduces the concentration of healthy compounds in the blood, especially vitamin C, vitamin D ...
- Causes the body to become desensitized to signals that tell the brain that you feel full or should reduce your appetite.
- Puts excess strain on the heart, other vital organs, and joints, which increases the chance that they will not work normally in the future.

And that is not all! Belly fat has been associated with the following conditions:

- Alzheimer's disease, dementia, and other neurological diseases
- Asthma—may cause increases in estradiol and IgE (so women may be more susceptible)
- Breathlessness
- Cancer (postmenopausal breast, cervical, colorectal, endometrial, gallbladder, kidney, and aggressive prostate cancer, to name just a few)
- Cataracts
- Cardiovascular disease (heart disease, heart failure, clots, strokes, atrial fibrillation, and sudden cardiac death)
- Diabetes
- Erectile dysfunction
- Female sexual dysfunction
- Fertility problems (polycystic ovary syndrome)
- Fetal problems (from maternal obesity)
- Gall bladder disease

- Gastroesophageal reflux disease (GERD) or heartburn
- Gout (high uric acid levels in the body)
- High blood pressure (hypertension)
- High cholesterol
- Kidney stones and kidney disease
- Lower back pain/problems
- Osteoarthritis (especially of the knee)
- Pregnancy complications (such as preeclampsia/high blood pressure)
- Respiratory problems
- Sleep apnea
- Surgical risk (especially with anesthesia)
- Urinary incontinence

Some things to remember:

- Pick a diet (or not) that lets you get 100 to 200 calories less per day, whether or not you want to believe that is what is going on ... in other words, perhaps being B.S.ed here is good!
- Never exercise excessively to lose weight, because this not only can reduce the effectiveness of your immune system but will also simply stimulate your hunger to a point where you will just eat more calories than usual and not be able to lose weight!
- The only way to reduce belly fat is to lose weight overall and continue lifting weights. Forget all those belly devices and all other quick-fix methods that claim they can reduce belly fat.
- If you are frustrated because you are not losing weight by exercising and eating better, please keep lifting weights, because that will help you to become more toned, increase your metabolism, and help to burn belly fat. You will look better, look more sexy, and feel better.

Dietary Supplements and Drugs

Most dietary supplements do *not* help cause significant weight loss, and some may be very dangerous for your heart and cardiovascular health.

- Bitter orange peel extract. This ingredient is common to many weight-loss dietary supplements. It works like ephedra because it is a stimulant, and it is not healthy in my opinion.

- Cinnamon powder or American ginseng supplements. Some believe there is good evidence that cinnamon (the spice) can help with weight loss, but again this is preliminary except for the evidence that it is heart healthy. A couple teaspoons a day may help, because cinnamon works similarly to a very small dose of a diabetic drug in that it helps increase the body's sensitivity to insulin. The problem is that taking too much can cause your blood sugar to drop quickly, and theoretically there is a chance you could pass out. This is similar to what has been seen in the past with American ginseng dietary supplements, so be aware that these may help a little, but also be careful!
- CLA (conjugated linoleic acid) seems to have a little research supporting it, but the long-term safety and real tangible effectiveness do not knock my socks off.
- Fiber pills. Do not take fiber pills because, in my opinion, they are a gigantic waste of your money! There are lots of cheap fiber options (fruits, veggies, beans, flaxseed, cereals ...) that work one hundred times better than the pills.
- Omega-3 dietary supplements (fish oil). New clinical research from Australia shows that combined with moderate exercise it may help accelerate weight loss more than exercise by itself. Ask your doctor if you can take 1 to 2 fish oil pills a day, along with your exercise routine, to improve your weight loss.
- Prescription drugs. Although weight-loss drugs may provide some help, they have not been effective long-term and certainly come with numerous side effects. Meridia® (sibutramine) is not bad, but it may increase your blood pressure. It is still the best and one of the only two FDA-approved prescription drugs for long-term weight loss.
- New over-the-counter drug. "Alli®" in my opinion is not worth the cost right now because it works by blocking the absorption of fat, including potentially some healthy fats. This means that the fat "shoots the tube." Alli is an old prescription drug that never worked that well. The company reduced the dosage, and now they sell it over the counter.
- Growth hormone (GH) or other hormones (B-HCG, testosterone in men ...) may help with weight loss, but the long-term heart-healthy safety issues of GH and B-HCG are still of concern.

Some drug companies are getting us excited about future weight-loss drugs in the pipeline, but I would tell you that most of what they are saying is B.S.! We went down this road recently with the drug Acomplia® (a drug that was supposed to be the next miracle weight-loss pill, and was even approved in some countries in Europe). It turned out to increase the risk of depression! If a weight-loss drug is clearly heart or mind unhealthy, then you should *not take it*!

Surgery and More

Liposuction does not cause healthy internal changes, which means that it can help you lose 10 to 20 pounds of fat quickly, but this is subcutaneous fat (right below the skin). For many people, cholesterol or heart disease risk does not change. So you may look better even though you may not live longer! In all seriousness, if you get liposuction, that is fine, but you should accept that it is for cosmetic reasons and not to improve your real internal health. One could argue that if you think you look better then you may start exercising more, and that thus the liposuction helped you a little. This is actually a weak argument offered by some B.S. experts. What I am seeing in some research and personal experience is that if a person looks to liposuction to stimulate a desire to exercise and eat better in general, it just may stimulate a desire instead to look to surgery to solve problems.

Gastric band and gastric bypass surgery may help a lot, but only a small number of individuals actually qualify for this procedure or surgery as a last resort. I do not want to B.S. you here; these procedures have been nothing short of a miracle for some patients. However, these procedures should also be an example to many people of how well your body responds to becoming more healthy, and I do not mean just from surgery, but in general.

These procedures have been shown in recent studies to significantly lower the risk of dying young from all causes, but they have also shown a higher rate of associated mental health issues. No one should have surgery for weight loss without having a psychological evaluation before and after the procedure. A small number of patients looking for a quick fix to their problems are at a higher risk of having mental health issues. To be safe rather than sorry, it makes complete sense to have your mental health evaluated before the procedure, right after the procedure, and continuing periodically long after the procedure has been completed. Patients who have had these surgeries will tell you that it is not easy having your stomach be the size of a baseball, because you can only eat certain foods in small pieces, and you have to consume a variety of nutritional supplements due to absorption issues. Oh, by the way, some of you have to do this every single day for the rest of your life! Ouch!

If you are one of those people who strictly determine their worth by stepping on a scale, well, let me give you a piece of advice—learn to live without the scale and throw the damn thing out! Otherwise, stepping on a weight scale that is on a balanced hard surface is best. If you step on a scale that is on a soft surface, this will artificially increase your weight reading on the scale.

Dr. Moyad, you make weight loss, at least at times in your book, sound simple, but I have bad genes or a slow metabolism, so what about people like me?

There is little doubt that some people have a slower metabolism compared to others because of age, genetics, hormones, lack of hormones, etc. However, you have to think of this like a car. Some of you are born like an expensive well-oiled machine that never needs much attention or service. Others are built like the cheapest car in the world that needs constant attention just to keep up on the road of life. The bottom line is that whether you are the low-maintenance or high-maintenance car may be out of your control, but can a high-maintenance or less efficient car go 200,000 miles and still look good? You're damn right it can, but it is going to require more work. We accept that fact in every other aspect of life, so why not with weight and metabolism?

Your Goal: Maintain a healthy weight, or at least try not to gain excess weight, especially around the waist, by both exercising and appreciating the "calorie." Learn how to reduce calories in general compared to being told to be obsessed with fats, proteins, or even the carbohydrate content of any food or beverage. Keep in mind that almost every fad diet ever invented operates on the concept of pulling back on about 100 to 200 calories per day to help with weight loss, regardless of whether you notice it or not. So, do what you need to do to cut back 100 to 200 calories a day, even if you have to B.S. yourself!

Step 13 around the B.S.—Fat Is Not Your Enemy

Please, pay attention to the types of fat in your diet. Increasing your intake of healthy fats and reducing your intake of some of the unhealthy fats make sense and are associated with a better quality of life This does not mean that you have to completely eliminate saturated fat intake!

> "If you have been good, you have earned the right to be bad once in a while."

> —Dr. Moyad, circa 1997
> when talking about things like saturated fat

| Dr. B.S.

"Low-fat diets are healthy!"

| Dr. Moyad's No B.S.

"Low-fat diets are outdated and simply make no sense for most of us today because the 'calorie' is now king or queen of your body. In general, you can eat everything but not a whole lot of anything!"

Research in the past has focused on lowering your overall fat intake in order to maintain a healthy body. Recently this has been challenged (thank goodness!). Controversy over this issue probably now exists because it is rather easy today to consume an excess of calories from fat, protein, or sugar. In the past, most calories came from fat. Today, portion sizes also have changed.

There are two types of fat with which you should be concerned—saturated fat, also known as "hydrogenated fat," and "trans fat," also known as "partially hydrogenated fat." Both of these types of fat have been linked to heart disease and cancer. Simply picking up several similar products and choosing the one that is lower in saturated and trans fat is the first step toward healthy eating. For example, when buying margarine, potato chips, or even cookies, try choosing the product that is lowest in saturated and trans fat, and also watch the calorie count. Choosing some of the more healthy fats, such as "monounsaturated" and "polyunsaturated" fats, is not only heart healthy, but also seems immune healthy.

Type of Dietary Fat	Where Is It Commonly Found?	Good or Bad Fat & Impact on Cholesterol vs. Carbohydrates (sugars)
Monounsaturated fat	Healthy plant-based cooking oils (canola, olive …), nuts	Good Lowers LDL & increases HDL
Polyunsaturated fat (includes omega-3 fatty acids)	Healthy plant-based cooking oils (canola, safflower, soybean …), flaxseed, fish, nuts, soybeans	Good Lowers LDL & increases HDL
Saturated fat (also known as hydrogenated fat)	Non-lean meat, high-fat dairy, some fast foods	Some are bad Increases LDL & increases HDL (note how it increases HDL … interesting, isn't it?)
Trans fat (also known as partially hydrogenated fat)	Some margarine, fast foods, snack foods, deep-fried foods	Bad Increases LDL & lowers HDL

Dr. Moyad, I am worried about trans fat? I have nightmares that it is coming to get me, so what should I do?

Nothing! That's right, nothing! Please accept that you cannot possibly worry about everything in this life or else you will have no time to enjoy anything. There are certain health issues where economic and public pressure alone will solve the problem for you (like reducing hormone levels in milk)! And this is one of those situations! This pressure is already having a huge impact on removing large amounts of these substances from our food. So relax and compare labels, and in general pick the product lower in trans fat, but soon there will not be much to compare to, so it's all going to be fine.

Dr. Moyad, I have still seen the words "does not contain trans fat" or "0 grams of trans fat" on the main label, but when I look at the smaller, harder-to-read ingredient label it states there is "partially hydrogenated vegetable oil." But that is the same thing as saying that it has trans fat, isn't it? So, is this false advertising?

Remember, I told you to chill out and relax! The reason you are seeing this is that you are still allowed to have less than 0.5 grams of trans fat per serving and say on the main label that you have no trans fat, and I agree with the FDA on this rule. So, this still means the product has a low amount of trans fat but not exactly zero, so follow the main label and relax. It is going to be okay, because the cost of going to zero trans fat across the board would not be worth it.

Again, calories are the concern and not just fat, protein, or sugar. Consuming smaller portion sizes is the first step toward controlling calories. If you are concerned about fat intake, choose items that are low in saturated and trans fat, and increase your intake of mono-unsaturated and polyunsaturated fat. However, do not be fooled because when I say pick healthier fats, I am saying just lower your overall intake of calories.

The enlargement of portion size creeps up on us from all directions. Keep in mind that sugary soda is only one of the many beverage or food products that you are exposed to on a regular basis. The problem of portion size is demonstrated in the table on soft drinks. I just bought popular cola drinks while I was working in Switzerland and in Korea, and the serving size was 8 ounces = 100 calories! That would never sell in the United States!

The Dr. Moyad History of Sugary Soda and the Ever-Increasing Serving Size

Years/Decades Dr. Moyad Wanted to Buy Soda with Sugar	Serving Size	Total Calories
1960s	8 ounces	100
1970s	12 ounces	150
1980s	16 ounces	200
1990s	20 ounces	250
2000 & beyond	24 ounces	300

So, is this next table a surprise? The average weight of children ages 12 to 17 has also increased with the portion sizes.

Gender	1966	Year 2000 to present
Boys	125 pounds	141 pounds
Girls	118 pounds	130 pounds

If you reduce your intake of saturated fat in general, you lower your intake of calories in general. For example, let's look at whole milk, 2%, 1%, and skim milk, and tell me what you notice.

Type of Milk	Saturated Fat in a Serving (8 ounces)	Total Calories in a Serving (8 ounces)
Almond milk	0 grams	40–60
Skim/Soy milk	0 grams	80
1% milk	1.5 grams	100
2% milk	3 grams	120
Whole milk	5 grams	150
Breast milk	5 grams	160
Goat's milk	6.5 grams	170
Buffalo milk	11.25 grams	235
Sheep's milk	11 grams	260
Reindeer milk	Does it really matter? Now you know why Santa Claus is obese.	580

Naturally, for most foods, if you increase the amount of fat or especially saturated fat, it also increases the total calories you ingest, as seen in the milk table. So, what is the bigger problem, saturated fat, or the calories, or both? It is difficult to say, because in the past most individuals who consumed high amounts of saturated fat or dairy products also consumed more calories than the average individual did. I am more worried about the total calories consumed rather than the saturated fat amount, but by lowering your saturated fat intake you can achieve two goals—lower fat and lower calories in your diet.

Some people believe that foods or beverages higher in saturated fat may make you feel full faster so that you do not consume more calories. Also, some types of saturated fat may actually increase your "good cholesterol" or HDL! Wow! For example, lauric acid (found in coconut) can increase HDL, but it can also increase LDL, and this is what makes some doctors nervous!

Let's look at some saturated fats and where they are found. For example, there is butyric acid (a saturated fat with 4 carbons) that is found in butter. And there is lauric acid, mentioned above, which is common not only in coconut oil but also in breast milk and palm oil and has 12 carbons. Myristic acid has 14 carbons and is found in dairy and cow's milk. Palmitic acid is a saturated fat with 16 carbons and is found in palm oil and meat. Stearic acid has 18 carbons and is found in cocoa butter and chocolate and in meat. So, let's take a look at the table and recognize that saturated fat is not necessarily a bad thing, because many healthy foods have a small quantity of it. Getting it in moderation is a natural part of a healthy diet. However, reducing your saturated fat intake is another simple way, in general, to reduce your overall caloric intake.

Approximate Saturated Fat as a Percentage of the Total Fat

Food	Lauric Acid (12-carbon saturated fat)	Myristic Acid (14-carbon saturated fat)	Palmitic Acid (16-carbon saturated fat)	Stearic Acid (18-carbon saturated fat)
Butter	5%	10%	30%	15%
Cashews	2%	1%	10%	5%
Coconut oil	45%	20%	10%	5%
Dark chocolate	0%	0%	35%	45%
Eggs	0%	0%	25%	10%
Ground beef	0%	5%	25%	15%
Salmon	0%	1%	30%	5%
Soybean oil	0%	0%	10%	5%

Getting some saturated fat in your diet is no big deal if your overall caloric intake is low and you are maintaining your healthy weight and the rest of your excellent cardiovascular numbers. It should be up to the individual to decide the best way to reduce overall caloric intake. My favorite way is just to cut back on calories and foods or beverages that have more saturated fat compared to a competitive and similar-tasting brand of the same product. For example, I prefer skim milk to whole milk, and this allows me to get fewer calories and less saturated fat.

At the same time, you should live a fun life! If you have been very good with your lifestyle and diet, you've earned the right to be bad. Once in a while, indulge yourself with your favorite food. To not allow yourself the pleasure of some saturated fat once in a while, well, I guess that is your choice, which only leaves more for me and the people I try to convince daily that moderation is not just the key to life but the only key that fits my door!

Dr. Moyad, what is more important, eating a lower number of calories, eating less, or not allowing yourself to gain weight by burning or exercising away the extra calories you eat?

I get this question all the time. Professional athletes, even the skinny ones, eat more calories than most people eat in a day just to maintain their weight, but they are still getting tons of calories. So is this healthy? Well, it is sort of like comparing an apple and a horse. The first goal is to *get fit*, and the second goal is to *maintain a healthy weight*! The third goal is to be able to *do all of this while getting a lower caloric intake*. Personally, I couldn't care less if the third goal is never met because you are one of the most amazing and highest paid athletes in the world! For example, the Olympic swimmer Michael Phelps eats 10,000 calories a day just to maintain his skinny frame of a body, but I would not classify him as unhealthy. However, if you are not Michael Phelps, please try to keep the three goals in mind.

Your Goal: Primary Moyad goal = get fit (look good, feel sexy, and feel happy). Secondary goal = lose or maintain weight (look even better, feel more sexy, and feel happier). Tertiary goal = lower caloric intake (look your best and feel your best).

Review

You should know your diet and lifestyle information by now, so if I ask you a couple questions from Part II, you can answer them as quickly as you could repeat the name and some lines of your favorite movie.

How many calories in one tiny little pound (0.5 kg)? _____

How many calories should be reduced per day in your weight-loss program in order to copy almost every successful dieting program in the world? _____

Name two benefits, apart from the obvious, that regular weight lifting will give you? _____

Name two benefits, apart from the obvious, that regular exercise will give you? _____

Jogging or running is the best form of exercise for you—true or false? _____

Now tell me why you should have answered false.
_____

Exercise is one of the best ways to reduce the risk of depression—true or false? _____

Have you talked to your employer about getting more exercise time? _____

If you had to choose a prescription drug right now to help you with weight loss, which one would it be besides sibutramine (Meridia)? _____ (trick question)

If you had to choose a dietary supplement to help you lose weight, you know you should first think about adding lots of dietary fiber (not a pill) to your diet, but adding the heart-healthy and brain-healthy supplement known as _____ oil may also help!

Part III

Dr. Moyad's Other No B.S. Dietary & Lifestyle Changes

I should have named this part "How to Again *Not* Have a Ridiculous and Unhealthy Obsession with Health That Many B.S. Experts Support," or maybe I should have named it "The Mostly Pill Free Zone, Continued."

Please remember: Heart Healthy = All Healthy
and Heart Unhealthy = All Unhealthy

Step 14 around the B.S.—Alcohol

All types of alcohol (beer, hard liquor, red wine, white wine) in moderation (about 1 drink a day for women and 1 to 2 drinks a day for men) may be healthy, but in excess all types of alcohol may be deadly! If you really think that one type of alcoholic drink is healthier or more detrimental than another, well, I have some swampland in Florida to sell you!

| Dr. B.S.

"Red wine is the healthiest type of alcohol for you, so you should drink red wine if you drink alcohol!" or "Darker beer has more antioxidants, so drink beer that is darker!"

| Dr. Moyad's No B.S.

"Red wine has never been proven to be healthier than any other type of alcoholic drink—this is all marketing spin! All forms of alcohol (beer, hard liquor, red wine, white wine) in moderation are equally healthy, and all forms of alcohol in excess are equally dangerous! Do not start drinking alcohol just for the health benefits because it is not worth it. If you are going to drink alcohol, pick the one that tastes the best to you."

It is scary how many health experts seem to recommend red wine for your health. What is this based on? I have no idea, because some of the largest studies that have objectively looked at this issue have not found an overall health difference between alcoholic beverages. Perhaps it is the fact that the word *polyphenols* is used a lot with red wine, but this does not mean there is a clinical difference between the types of drinks consumed. B.S. experts like to use a lot of difficult sounding medical or scientific vernacular to increase their credibility, but most of this talk is simply B.S.!

I can easily create a marketing argument that beer is the healthiest alcohol product. For example, beer contains many antioxidants such as xanthohumol (hops used as a bittering agent in beer contain this unique flavonoid in small concentrations), which is associated with some positive laboratory studies against breast, colon, ovarian, and prostate cancer. Most beer also comes from fermented wheat juice, which contains antioxidants, but darker beers have more than the pale ales (like the chocolate situation). But who cares—drink the kind that tastes the best to you. Beer production uses the husk of the grain, which contributes a highly absorbable form of bone-building silicon called "silicate." This is why some studies have found that beer also may improve bone health.

In the Western world, one of the major sources of bio-available and bioactive silicon is beer. This is nice to know for the moderate beer drinkers of the world (like myself). If some beers in the future are made from oats and not barley, you may get beta-glucans, which may lower LDL (bad cholesterol) and provide a partial immune boost. Beer in some studies has also been associated with a lower risk of bladder cancer, but this is unproven as fluid consumption in general has been associated with a lower risk of bladder cancer.

I think you get the idea here that, depending on the way you spin things, one type of alcohol can look better than another. Some past studies on alcohol have been biased against beer drinkers, because on average wine drinkers in some countries were more likely to exercise and eat right while beer drinkers were more likely to be sedentary and not eat right. In other words, it was not the beer itself that was necessarily the problem, but the overall behavior of the average beer drinker.

Let's review a *serving* of alcohol, and what that means, and what is moderation, which to me has not changed and *will not change in my lifetime.*

- One serving of beer = 12 ounces (about 13.2 grams of alcohol).
- One serving of hard alcohol = 1.5-ounce shot of 80 proof liquor (15.1 grams of alcohol).
- One serving of wine = 4–6 ounces (about 10.8 to 15 grams of alcohol).
- 1 gram of alcohol = about 7 calories.

Now, it is important to understand daily moderate amounts of alcohol for women, which is about one serving a day, and for men it is one to two servings of alcohol per day. That is really it! Now, what does this actually mean? If you do not drink from Monday to Saturday, this does *not* mean that you can drink 7 servings on Sunday if you are a woman or 14 servings on Sunday if you are a man.

Now, let's review what alcohol in moderation may do for you.

- Increase good cholesterol or HDL
- Improve bone health (that's right, regardless of what the B.S. experts say)
- Reduce your risk of a heart attack or stroke (may thin your blood or reduce stickiness of clot-forming platelets, reduce fibrinogen)
- Improve mental health
- May improve sexual function (controversial)

Alcohol in excess can cause many problems, including:

- Increases triglycerides
- Increases sugar levels
- Increases the risk of osteoporosis
- Adds a large source of calories (meaning you gain a lot of weight)
- Increases blood pressure
- Damages the heart
- Suppresses the immune system
- Reduces folic acid concentrations and a variety of other nutrients
- Increases the risk of some cancers—oral/esophageal and breast cancer and possibly many other cancers such as lung cancer.
- Reduces sexual performance

Alcohol contains plant estrogens such as resveratrol in wine, which is why in moderation it may improve bone health. This substance also explains why alcohol may increase the risk of breast cancer. Alcohol also reduces folic acid, which is why some respectable health experts believe that if you drink alcohol in moderation you should get a daily cheap multivitamin with at least 400 micrograms of folic acid. This makes sense, but keep in mind that even moderate drinking can reduce your blood level of all kinds of wonderful vitamins and minerals, including vitamin C.

Drinking grape juice does not necessarily replace alcohol's benefits. Grape juice does not raise your good cholesterol as well as alcohol. Grape juice in excess is high in calories, just like alcohol.

Your Goal: Drink alcohol in moderation only or do not drink at all.

Step 15 around the B.S.—Fiber

Fiber is the best natural internal anti-aging product ever invented. Consume more total dietary fiber (about 20–40 grams/day) from food and even from low-calorie fiber bars for overall health advantages. Soluble and insoluble fibers are both beneficial, but getting more insoluble fiber provides more benefits. Fiber pills are B.S., because you need to take 35 to 75 pills a day to reach the recommended daily amount of fiber ... no thanks. Most fiber bars are B.S. because they are either too expensive, low in calories with little to no fiber, high in calories with little fiber or some fiber, high in calories with a moderate amount of fiber, or high in just soluble fiber, and almost all contain the wrong ratio, amounts, or even types of fiber! Also, keep in mind simplicity ... just *one bowl* of All-Bran® Buds or Fiber-One® or another cereal with a lot of insoluble fiber (10 grams or more) with several tablespoons of ground flaxseed or another high-fiber product that can be cheaply added on the cereal equals almost 20 grams of fiber. Wow! The government and other official groups have good intentions when they recommend lots of fiber, but they are not guiding us to realistic, practical, and moderate fiber sources that can be included in our lifestyles.

> "As I got older I began to quickly notice that at some point my wild oats began to change into All-Bran®."
>
> —Anonymous, circa 2006. I saw this sign at a truck stop in California.

| Dr. B.S.

"Fiber does *not* reduce your risk of colon cancer!"

| Dr. Moyad's No B.S.

"Whatever! Who gives a _____ (beep)? Pass the All-Bran, Slimming Squares, soy milk or whatever milk, and doughnuts and leave me alone! You find me a dietary supplement or drug that has all the benefits of fiber and I will give you a Nobel Prize for that drug, but you will never find a drug with all the benefits of fiber."

Many foods contain a high amount of fiber, including beans, fruits, vegetables, flaxseed, whole grains, oats ... Keep in mind that if you increase your intake of fiber, you should also increase your consumption of water.

Listed here is part of the Moyad List of Fiber Benefits.

- Helps with weight control because it delays the emptying of gastric contents, delays the absorption of fats, and promotes a feeling of fullness.
- Improves glucose or sugar balance by delaying the movement and absorption of carbohydrates into the small intestine, so you simply burn your dietary fuel more efficiently and evenly.
- Reduces cholesterol levels by binding with bile (cholesterol-carrying products) in the intestine and causing it to be excreted or eliminated.
- Increases the weight of the stool and softens the stool to promote regular and smooth bowel movements.
- Reduces the colon transit time so that the stool goes through intestines faster.
- Reduces pressure within the colon.
- Reduces the risk of cancer? Maybe, but who cares! Look at all the other benefits!
- Reduces the risk of diverticulitis (It is called "left-side appendicitis" for a reason, and it is very common as we get older ... ouch!)
- Reduces symptoms of irritable bowel syndrome (IBS).
- Reduces the risk of and may even treat hemorrhoids or constipation.
- Reduces the risk of gastroesophageal reflux disease (GERD).
- Reduces blood pressure.
- May reduce the risk of preeclampsia, which is a potentially life-threatening blood pressure problem in pregnancy.
- May reduce a man's PSA blood test number by lowering cholesterol.
- Acts as a prebiotic to promote higher amounts of friendly bacteria in your colon to improve overall digestive health.

Fun Facts about Fiber

- Human digestive enzymes cannot break down fiber.
- Soluble and insoluble fiber were given different names to reflect their ability to dissolve in water.
- Soluble fiber is now also known as "viscous fiber" on some labels.

- Soluble fiber causes excess gas production in the bowel, while insoluble fiber, in general, does not. This is because the bacteria in your gastrointestinal tract can break down soluble fiber and can produce a lot of gas and bloating.
- Dietary fiber is actually considered a complex carbohydrate.
- Some low-carbohydrate diets allow you to subtract the dietary fiber amount from the total carbohydrate amount before adding your total daily intake of carbs (most low-carb diets follow this rule).
- Fiber powdered supplements (I hate them) usually need to be taken with a glass of water to reduce the risk of impaction or blockage of a part of the bowel, which can be a medical emergency.
- Fiber supplements (I hate them) especially should not be taken at the same time as prescription medications (wait 1 to 2 hours before or after) because it can reduce their absorption.
- Some types of dietary fiber contain a compound called phytate (also known as inositol hexaphosphate) that may form insoluble complexes with some nutrients and reduce their absorption, but only when fiber is consumed in excessive quantities that would never allow you to leave your home (let alone the bathroom).

Now let's learn about why both soluble and insoluble fibers are important.

The Specific Benefits of Soluble and Insoluble Fiber

Benefit	Soluble Fiber	Insoluble Fiber
Lowers total cholesterol & bad (LDL) cholesterol and reduces blood pressure	Yes	Maybe
Reduces sugar or glucose blood levels after a meal	Yes	No
Reduces the absorption of sugar or glucose from the small intestine	Yes	No
Delays gastric emptying or increases the amount of time it takes for food to leave the stomach, thus giving a sense of fullness & discouraging higher caloric intakes	Yes	No

Increases the production of intestinal gas	Yes	No
Increases the speed at which the stool moves through the intestines, reducing the impact time that carcinogens have on the intestine	Yes	Yes
Increases the size of the stool & the frequency of bowel movements	Yes	Yes
Reduces the amount of essential nutrients absorbed by the body	No (not in moderation)	No (not in moderation)

Healthy foods in general contain the perfect quality (notice I did not say quantity) of fiber. So let's learn where you can find this amazing ingredient! However, always keep in mind the overall calorie count because there are a few high-calorie high-fiber foods. Comparing labels is the way to go here!

Dietary Fiber in Some Fruits (per serving size)	Amount of Fiber (in grams)
Dried plums or prunes (3)	6
Apple with skin (1)	3–3.5
Pear with skin (½)	3
Prunes (3)	3
Raisins (¼ cup)	3
Raspberries (½ cup)	3
Strawberries (1 cup)	3
Banana (1)	2.5
Orange (1)	2.5
Peach with skin (1)	2
Tomato (1)	1.5–2.5
Grapefruit (½)	1.5
Cherries (5)	1–1.5

Dietary Fiber in Some Vegetables (per serving size)	Amount of Fiber (in grams)
Artichoke (cooked)	10 (1 medium-size artichoke) 7 (1 cup of artichoke hearts)
Parsnips (1 cup)	5.5
Broccoli (1 cup)	4.5
Brussels sprouts (1 cup)	4.5
Sweet potatoes (1)	3.5
Zucchini (1 cup)	3.5
Green beans (1 cup)	3
Red cabbage (1 cup)	3
Corn (½ cup)	3
Kale (1 cup)	3
Carrot (raw or cooked) (1 cup)	2–4.5
Spinach (1 cup)	2–4
Cauliflower (1 cup)	2–2.5
Asparagus (1 cup)	2
Potato (1)	1.5 and 2.5
Bean sprouts (½ cup)	1.5
Mushrooms (½ cup)	1.5
Celery (½ cup)	1
Lettuce (1 cup)	1
Cucumber (½ cup)	0.5
Green pepper (½ cup)	0.5

Dietary Fiber in Some Legumes/Beans (per serving size)	Amount of Fiber (in grams)
Cranberry beans (⅔ cup)	12
Baked beans (½ cup)	9

Kidney beans (½ cup cooked)	7–8
Navy beans (½ cup cooked)	6
Lima beans (½ cup cooked)	4.5
Dried peas (½ cup cooked)	4–5
Lentils (½ cup cooked)	4–5
Split peas (½ cup)	6.7

Notice in the next table how food label comparison while you are shopping is critical. For example, if you buy regular spaghetti you would be lucky to get any fiber, but by comparing it to a whole wheat spaghetti you do not necessarily get a lot more calories but you get a lot more fiber.

Dietary Fiber in Some Grains/Cereals (per serving size)	Amount of Fiber (in grams)
Wheat-bran cereal (All-Bran, FiberOne®) (⅓ cup)	10–14
Oatmeal (¾ cup)	4–5
Bran Chex® cereal (⅔ cup)	4.5
Raisin bran–type cereals (⅔ cup)	4
Spaghetti (whole wheat) (½ cup cooked)	4–6
Whole-wheat bread (1 slice)	2–3
Bran muffins (1)	2.5
Shredded wheat cereal (⅔ cup)	2.5
Rye crisp bread (1 slice)	2
Grape-Nuts® cereal (¼ cup)	1.5
Brown rice (½ cup cooked)	1–1.5
Spaghetti (regular) (½ cup cooked)	1
White bread (1 slice)	0.5
Corn flakes cereal (1¼ cup)	0.5
White rice (½ cup cooked)	0–0.2

Dietary Fiber in Some Nuts/Seeds (per serving size)	Amount of Fiber (in grams)
Chestnuts (10 roasted kernels)	4–5
Flaxseed (golden) (2 Tbsp.)	4–6
Flaxseed (regular, brown) (2 Tbsp.)	3–4
Almonds (5 nuts)	3–4
Sunflower seeds (1 oz.)	3–4
Brazil nuts (1 oz.)	2–3
Hazelnuts (filberts) (10 nuts, raw)	1–2
Macadamia nuts (1 oz.)	2–3
Pistachio nuts (1 oz.)	2–3
Peanuts (1 oz. raw)	2–3
Pecans (1 oz.)	2–3
Walnuts (¼ cup)	2–3
Cashews (1 oz. raw)	1–2
Sesame seeds (2 Tbsp.)	1–2
Squash seeds (1 oz., dried)	1–2
Pine nuts (1 oz.)	1
Pumpkin seeds (1 oz., dried)	0–1

The key to taking advantage of fiber is to locate foods that are high in fiber and lower in calories. Compare labels!

Many prestigious medical organizations have wonderful dietary recommendations *except* when it comes to fiber, because many of them will recommend 20–30 grams of fiber a day. They recommend that most of this should be soluble (viscous) fiber, but *I could not disagree more*.

You need to get as much insoluble fiber as possible, which is similar to how nature set up its internal content of fiber in all sorts of fruits and vegetables. The simplest way to do this is to eat a cereal in the morning and add flaxseed, small fruits, or other simple fiber sources (oat bran) to it. For example, my bran cereal gives me 13 to 15 grams of fiber per bowl. I add several tablespoons of flaxseed and I have almost *20 grams of fiber in one meal*. I have almost reached my daily requirement in just one bowl of cereal! For the rest of the day, you can get some fiber from some fruits and vegetables, bean products, nuts and seeds, whole grains, and even fiber bars (Slimming Squares). However, look for the fiber bar that is lowest in calories and higher in insoluble fiber.

Note: Chia seeds (not the old funny TV commercial) are a new source and one of the largest sources of plant fiber and plant omega-3 fatty acids ever discovered! Look for them at a health food or grocery store near you!

Your Goal: Include 25 to 30 grams of fiber in my daily diet (mostly insoluble fiber).

Step 16 around the B.S.—Fish & Other Sources of Omega-3 Fatty Acids

| Dr. B.S.

"Salmon is the healthiest fish to eat, because it is best for your heart, skin, and the rest of your body!"

| Dr. Moyad's No B.S.

"Whatever! Many types of fish are healthy, including salmon, but I find it very interesting that most fish oils sold around the world and used in successful clinical trials of fish oil come from anchovies and sardines! Regardless of what the B.S. experts are telling you, plant sources of omega-3 fatty acids are just as important as those from fish. However, always keep in mind the risk-to-benefit ratio of any product, and that is why eating small- to moderate-sized oily fish will always make sense for people who like to eat fish (yes, including pregnant women)."

Omega-3 and omega-6 fatty acids are essential fatty acids, which means that they are essential to human health but cannot be made in the body. For this reason, they must come from diet.

There are three omega-3 fatty acids or essential fatty acids that you need to know about for now. The first is ALA (alpha-linolenic acid), and it comes from a variety of foods, especially flaxseed, nuts (walnuts), and vegetable oils (canola, soybean), but not from fish. The other two are known as EPA (eicosapentaenoic acid) and DHA (docosahexaenoic acid), and these come mostly from fish and fish oils.

Sources of ALA (Plant Omega-3)

Food	ALA (plant omega-3) Content in 1–2 Tablespoons
Flaxseed (linseed) oil	8.5 grams
Flaxseed (ground)	2.2 grams (2,200 mg!)
Walnut oil	1.4 grams
Canola oil	1.3 grams

Soybean oil	0.9 grams
Walnuts (English)	0.7 grams
Olive oil	0.1 grams

ALA is a source of calories and energy for humans, and it can be made into EPA and DHA by the human body. However, contrary to popular past belief, only a small percentage of ALA is actually made into EPA and DHA by the body (only about 1–10 percent into EPA on a good day, and very little ALA is made into DHA at all). This is probably because ALA is quickly used as an energy source for the body. Thus, in order to get a diversity of omega-3 into the body, you have to not only consume fish and fish oil, but food and oil sources of ALA. You cannot consume ALA alone or EPA and DHA alone—you need a diverse diet.

Omega-6 fatty acids are easier to get in the American diet. Vegetable oils, meat, and several plant-based oils (evening primrose, borage oil, and black currant) contain omega-6 fatty acids. The point is that the typical unhealthy American diet contains higher concentrations of omega-6 compounds and lower amounts of omega-3 compounds. One good theory as to why some healthy populations live longer is that the ratio of omega-6 to omega-3 fatty acids in their diet is almost equal (about 1:1), but in the American diet the ratio of omega-6 to omega-3 is too high (ranging from 10:1 to 15:1). One goal is to change the intake to reflect those of healthier populations.

I am not implying that omega-6 fatty acids are unhealthy, because they are not, contrary to what some authors claim. It is just that we are getting too much omega-6 from unhealthy sources (fast food, fried food) and not enough omega-3 from healthy sources. The American diet with its 10 to 15:1 ratio of omega-6 to omega-3 fatty acids does not compare well with the heart-healthy Mediterranean or Japanese regions (2:1 ratio). The ideal situation is a 1:1 ratio.

The goal is to consume more ALA, EPA, and DHA. Do not be B.S.ed by certain companies that tell you that one type of omega-3 is definitely healthier than another type. All are healthy—for example, DHA may be better for the baby's brain and eye development, but EPA seems to do a better job of reducing the risk of depression. EPA and DHA are heart healthy, but ALA also helps to maintain heart health.

EPA and DHA are polyunsaturated fatty acids that are found mostly in seafood. The oilier the fish, the more EPA and DHA they usually contain. For example, high concentrations are found in anchovies, herring, mackerel, sardines, salmon, and tuna. All fish contain EPA and DHA, but the amount varies among fish and within the same species of fish, depending on environmental and seasonal factors and whether the fish are farm- or wild-raised. For example, farm-raised catfish usually have less EPA and DHA than wild catfish, but farm-raised salmon and trout usually have similar amounts to the wild form.

Recently researchers have found that some types of fungus and algae contain DHA, and in some cases these sources have been cultivated and commercialized, mostly to supply the infant formula and maternal and child health industry. They also are becoming popular as supplements, and these products will be discussed more in the section on pills.

There are so many human studies now that have shown that consuming healthy foods high in ALA, EPA, and DHA is not only heart healthy but, you guessed it, mostly all healthy, that it just makes sense to consume more.

Here is a list of some mechanisms by which omega-3 fatty acids may be reducing the risk of cardiovascular disease (CVD). Some of these benefits have also been found for omega-3 pills (see omega-3 pill in the section on pills).

- Reduces the chance of your heart beating in an abnormal way (may reduce ventricular arrhythmia)
- Reduces heart rate and blood pressure
- Reduces fasting and after-meal triglycerides (may also slightly improve HDL or good cholesterol)
- Reduces the size and vulnerability of plaques that block arteries
- Increases the size or relaxes blood vessels (promotes nitric oxide–induced endothelial relaxation)
- Makes platelets or clotting less likely to occur

There have been some recent health concerns that eating fish may also expose you to a number of unhealthy compounds that have accumulated in some fish more than others. The biggest concern about eating fish today is that they may be contaminated with a variety of compounds from the environment, especially methylmercury. In general, smaller fish have less mercury compared to older, larger predatory fish. The FDA is concerned about the following fish being consumed during pregnancy: king mackerel, shark, swordfish, tilefish (also known as golden bass or golden snapper), and even non-light tuna.

In the lists below, you will notice how the fish with lower mercury levels are the smaller oily fish in general, which is exactly from where most fish oil pills come, so that is the good news!

Fish/Shellfish with Low Levels of Mercury

Anchovies	Hake	Scallops
Butterfish	Herring	Shad
Calamari	Lobster (rock/spiny)	Shrimp
Catfish	Mackerel	Sole
Caviar (farmed)	Oysters	Sturgeon
Clams	Perch (saltwater/	Tilapia
Cod	ocean)	Trout (farmed
Crab (king)	Pollock	or freshwater
Crawfish/crayfish	Salmon (farmed or	& rainbow)
Flounder	wild)	Tuna (light canned)
Haddock	Sardines	Whitefish

Fish/Shellfish with Medium Levels of Mercury

Bass (lake)	Mahimahi	Snapper
Carp	Perch (freshwater)	Tuna (fresh Pacific
Crab (blue,	Rock cod	albacore)
Dungeness, snow)	Skate	

Fish/Shellfish with High Levels of Mercury

Amberjack	King mackerel	Shark
Bass (saltwater)	Lobster (Maine)	Swordfish
Bluefish	Marlin	Tilefish
Croaker	Orange roughy	Tuna (ahi, fresh
Grouper	Sea Trout	bluefin, white
Halibut		albacore)

It must be recognized that the EPA's safe mercury dose is based on inappropriate studies of people who consume mostly whale meat and blubber containing multiple chemicals—PCBs, cadmium, pesticides, persistent organic pollutants, DDT, etc.—of which mercury is only one of the many troublesome compounds. One of the largest studies of fish consumption in the world was published in the *Lancet* recently and found that pregnant women with a lower intake of fish during pregnancy were at a higher risk of giving birth to a child with developmental problems. Eating fish 2–3 times a week in pregnancy was associated with the lowest risk of developmental problems.

Both wild fish and farmed fish are good sources of omega-3. Farmed fish are fed products that contain fish protein and fish oil, and this is why farmed fish also contain omega-3 fatty acids. Wild fish actually have a slightly more unpredictable amount of omega-3 because the amount depends on the maturity of the fish and when it is caught. It should be kept in mind that the positives still outweigh the negatives here for farmed fish. In other words, the amount of contaminants in farmed fish is usually low, and it is still better to eat these fish compared to not eating fish at all for your health. Eating commercially prepared *fried fish* (restaurants, fast food, frozen) should be discouraged or minimized as it provides no health benefit and is low in omega-3 and high in trans fat.

Recent studies of farm-raised fish (such as salmon) have shown that they can contain as much as 50 to 75 percent less vitamin D compared to wild fish. Some farm-raised salmon also have vitamin D2, whereas the more natural vitamin D3 is found in wild salmon. The cause of this difference requires further investigation, but the vitamin D content in healthy farm-raised fish is still good.

The following table gives the approximate omega-3 oil concentrations from a partial group of fish and shellfish, listed in alphabetical order, and how many servings a week would give you the government recommended weekly intake (1,750 to 3,500 mg) to protect your heart with the healthy benefits of fish! Compare this with most dietary supplements where you need seven capsules per week or one per day to equal your minimum intake of fish oil for proper heart health.

Fish/Shellfish*	Omega-3 Total Amount (EPA + DHA) in 1 Serving (approximate)	Servings/Week to Meet Total Omega-3 Recommended Daily Allowance
Anchovy*	1,165 mg	2
Catfish (farmed)	250 mg	7
Catfish (wild)	350 mg	5
Clams	240 mg	7
Cod (Atlantic)	285 mg	7
Cod (Pacific)	435 mg	4

Crab (Alaskan king)	350 mg	5
Fish sandwich (fast food)	335 mg	5
Fish sticks (frozen)	195 mg	9
Flounder/Sole	500 mg	4
Halibut	740 mg	3 (high in mercury)
Haddock	200 mg	9
Herring* (Atlantic or Pacific)	1 710 mg	1
King mackerel	620 mg	3 (high in mercury)
Lobster	70 mg	25
Mackerel (Atlantic)*	1060 mg	2
Mahimahi	220 mg	8
Mussels	665 mg	3
Oysters (Eastern, farmed, Pacific)	585 mg	3
Pollock (Alaskan)	280 mg	7
Salmon (farmed)* All types of salmon	4,500 mg	Less than 1
Salmon (wild)* All types of salmon	1,775 mg	1 (high in vitamin D3)
Sardines*	555 mg	3
Scallops	310 mg	6
Shrimp	265 mg	7
Shark	585 mg	3 (but high in mercury)
Snapper*	545 mg	3
Swordfish	870 mg	2 (but high in mercury)
Tilapia	100–150 mg	20
Tilefish or golden bass	1,360 mg	2 (high in mercury)
Trout* (rainbow, farmed, or wild)	580 to 800 mg	3

(continued)

Fish/Shellfish*	Omega-3 Total Amount (EPA + DHA) in 1 Serving (approximate)	Servings/Week to Meet Total Omega-3 Recommended Daily Allowance
Tuna (fresh)	900 mg	2 (moderate to high in mercury)
Tuna (light, skipjack)	230 mg	8
Tuna (white, albacore)	735 mg	3 (high in mercury)

*Fish in bold are moderate, practical, and generally safe to eat to get your recommended daily allowance of fish oil for heart health. It's OK to deviate several times a month, like eating halibut or regular tuna, because they are high in omega-3.

Also, there is recent research to suggest that the high amount of selenium in fish protects the fish and humans against the toxicity of mercury (accumulating in tissues of the body). It is possible that if you get the recommended daily allowance or less of selenium (around 70 mcg or less) in your multivitamin, this protects you from some of the mercury in fish.

Your Goal: For you and your children, eat fish that you like, that fit your budget, and that have a high content of omega-3 and in general have a low content of mercury.

Step 17 around the B.S.—Fruits & Vegetables

| Dr. B.S.

"Eat more fruits and vegetables, up to 9 to 10 servings a day for better health. And, pick the fruits and vegetables with the most color because they have the highest amount of antioxidants!"

| Dr. Moyad's No B.S.

"Try to eat a variety of fruits and vegetables every day or every few days, but pick the ones that you like to eat because the color does not matter as much as the importance of just including some in your diet. Keep in mind that the dull-colored fruits and vegetables are just as important as the bright-colored ones.

"What fruit or vegetable has the highest concentration of lycopene?"
The answer is watermelon! Congratulations; if you thought at one time it was a tomato, you were probably one of the many that were impacted by effective marketing.

Which fruit or vegetable has been *clearly* shown to reduce the risk of breast or prostate cancer?
The answer is none of them! Effective marketing campaigns strike again! Eat them in moderation because they are healthy and may reduce the risk of cardiovascular disease. And, if you eat some fruits and veggies, you are probably not eating a quadruple cheeseburger at the same time.

Fruits and vegetables contain many antioxidants and a lot of other so-called anti–heart disease and anti-cancer compounds. In the past, there was a focus on the compound found in tomatoes called lycopene for prostate and heart health. However, recent research has focused on a variety of fruits and vegetables and the potential benefits of each for health. Also, increasing your intake of a *variety* of fruits and vegetables will also keep you interested in eating these foods. For example, at our house we like to eat blueberries one day, strawberries on another, broccoli on another, watermelon on another, tomatoes on another, celery with some peanut butter on another, and so on. If we just ate tomatoes every day, we would get sick of them in just a few days.

Superfoods? Rainbow? Eat the bright color? *All of the fruits and vegetables have value!* In the largest and most comprehensive worldwide study of lifestyle and heart disease prevention (known as the 52 countries study), eating fruits and veggies daily was associated with a reduced risk of heart disease. The type of fruit and vegetable did not matter, nor did eating 30 servings a day matter. What really mattered was whether or not individuals *ate one or more servings of fruit and vegetables daily.*

What about the ORAC (Oxygen Radical Absorbance Capacity) value? I heard that fruits and vegetables with larger ORAC values are healthier for you? Is that true?

No. This value is determined in a laboratory and is supposed to impress you. Keep in mind that despite being impressive it does not imply clinically that one fruit or vegetable is healthier for you.

Cooked or raw fruits and vegetables—which one is better?

Who gives a damn? Eat it the way you like it. If you want to know, both are fine and healthy. Cooking reduces some nutrient content, but who cares? However, cooking can also release locked nutrients for better absorption. Cooking tomatoes unlocks lycopene. Cooking carrots or spinach increases the absorption of beta-carotene. Broccoli that is raw has more vitamins (like vitamin C), but cooking it allows more availability of anti-disease compounds. Cooking also creates more nutrient dense benefits compared to raw, because cooking shrinks the food into a smaller overall space and reduces the risk of gas and stomach upset and even infection that can occur with some raw products.

Are fast-food salads unhealthy?

No. Bagged lettuce and fast-food salads are safe. Fast-food salads are as safe as any fruit and vegetable in the grocery store. Fast-food companies buy produce from the same places as the grocery stores. Salads are washed thoroughly to remove compounds that can spoil them quickly, kept refrigerated, and served as fast as possible (within about 7–10 days). Salad greens are usually washed in a very lightly chlorinated wash/bath and rinsed again. The light chlorinated bath is critical to prevent food-borne illness. It removes any residues from the field, such as pesticides and fertilizers. It is safe, and this is also why some experts believe bagged lettuce is healthier compared to just a head of lettuce at the store (cleaned only on the outside).

I heard the peel of the fruit is healthy?

Yes! Researchers have long known that the peel of many fruits contains numerous nutrients and potential anti-disease compounds such as limonoids. Despite laboratory and test tube data, more research is needed in humans. In the meantime, I believe in the power of the peel. When you hear that fruits and vegetables are healthy, it also means that this may include the peel. Again, do researchers have strong proof that peels prevent disease?—no! However, this is one that just makes sense. Remove the peel of the apple, carrot, or cucumber, and you are removing some of the most important nutrients and fiber!

Your Goal: Eat a variety of fruits and vegetables, and not just tomatoes, pomegranates, or whatever other specific fruit or vegetable du jour is getting all of the commercial and marketing time and attention right now. And never be impressed by the antioxidant amount or value of a fruit or vegetable. All fruits and vegetables, regardless of their color, have something to offer or their own unique healthy components that need to be appreciated. All fruits and vegetables have some research to suggest they have anti-cancer and, more importantly, anti–heart disease properties.

**Please remember: Heart Healthy = All Healthy
and Heart Unhealthy = All Unhealthy!**

Step 18 around the B.S.—Fruit Juices & Other High-Calorie Beverages

Be careful about many fruit and vegetable juices and especially the exotic fruit drinks! You want more antioxidants, well, say hello to more calories and/or higher prices in many cases. Some of the so-called healthiest juices are actually unhealthy above moderate levels (more than 8 ounces a day) because they contain too many calories, and that can ultimately make you obese and unhealthy. Notice from the table below how most fruit and exotic juices have as many or more calories than a cola or beer.

Beverage Calories

Beverage	Approximate Calories (8 oz. serving)
Mixed fruit smoothie	200–250
Acai juice	150–200
Grape juice	170–180
Pomegranate juice	140–160
Pineapple juice or cherry juice	130–150
Orange, grapefruit, or apple juices or lemonade	100–120
Beer/wine/hard liquor	100–150
Watermelon juice	100–110
Cola and other soft drinks	100
Skim or soy milk	80–100
Carrot juice	70–80
Cranberry juice	70–80
Light beer	70–80
Blueberry juice	50–60
Gatorade® sports drink	50
Tomato juice or mixed vegetable tomato-based juice (V-8® …)	50
Coffee (with fat-free milk to cream)	5–50

Tea (black, green, Oolong…)	0-5
Diet soft drink	0
Water	0

Your Goal: Be aware of the calories in beverages.

**Please remember: Heart Healthy = All Healthy
and Heart Unhealthy = All Unhealthy!**

Step 19 around the B.S.—Nuts & Seeds and Learning the Moyad Healthy Fat Ratio

Nuts and seeds of all types are healthy and a perfect snack in moderation (a handful a day). They taste good, keep you heart healthy, and make you feel full so you eat less (lots of protein). But don't be fooled, because like many things healthy they can also have a lot of calories (about 5–10 calories per single piece of nut). If in doubt when comparing labels, add the monounsaturated + polyunsaturated fat amount and compare this total to the saturated fat amount. I call it the Moyad Healthy Fat Ratio or No B.S. ratio. The greater the ratio (for example, 12:1 is better than 5:1), the healthier the product in general when it comes to many dairy products, fish, meats, nuts, oils, and seeds. When comparing two similar products, it is a good way to decide the healthier product between the two.

Going nuts is good for you?

Most nuts are high in vitamins like vitamin E, high in other antioxidants, low in saturated fat, and high in monounsaturated fat, and some even contain omega-3 fatty acids. It is interesting that nuts such as walnuts, almonds, pistachios, Brazil nuts, and others have been associated with a lower risk of sudden cardiac death, and that they contain compounds associated with breast, colon, and prostate health. For example, Brazil nuts are one of the largest natural sources of selenium, and other nuts are some of the largest natural sources of vitamin E.

No B.S. Fast Facts on Nuts

- Seem to reduce the risk of sudden cardiac death, so this is reason enough to learn about them!
- Make you feel full so can help you lose weight
- Keep blood sugar levels normal
- Impact your cholesterol level in a healthy way
- Contains gamma-tocopherol or natural vitamin E that has been found to be potentially heart healthy.

Some of the Many Healthy Components of Nuts

- Copper (about 15–20 percent of your daily needs in one serving)

- Fiber (about 3 grams per serving, and 25 percent of the fiber is soluble)
- Folic acid (about 15 percent of your daily needs in one serving)
- Low to zero cholesterol
- Low in saturated fat
- Magnesium
- Monounsaturated fat (like oleic acid commonly found in olive oil)
- No trans fats in general
- Omega-3 and omega-6 healthy balance (polyunsaturated fats)
- Plant protein (amino acids like arginine)
- Plant sterols (like sitosterol found in cholesterol-lowering products)
- Potassium
- Resveratrol (a polyphenol compound in peanuts and grape skins)
- Vitamin E (gamma-tocopherol, the healthy kind of vitamin E)

Now, as with fruits and vegetables, I am going to quickly show you why eating a handful of nuts almost every day, regardless of the type, is smart, and do not be B.S.ed into believing that one nut is better than another. Before we start, it is important to understand the Moyad Healthy Fat Ratio. Add up the monounsaturated and polyunsaturated fat, and compare it to the saturated fat and calculate the ratio. The higher the ratio, the healthier a product is when comparing labels at the grocery store.

Some Nuts and Seeds (Serving = 1 ounce or 1/4 cup = 150–200 calories)	Nutrition and Moyad Fat Ratio
Almonds (170 calories)	High in monounsaturated fat (10 g) Polyunsaturated fat (4 g) Saturated fat (1 g) Moyad fat ratio 14:1 High in potassium (210 mg), fiber (3 g) & vitamin E
Brazil nuts (190 calories)	Monounsaturated fat (7 g) Polyunsaturated fat (21 g)

Some Nuts and Seeds (Serving = 1 ounce or 1/4 cup = 150–200 calories)	Nutrition and Moyad Fat Ratio
Brazil nuts (con't.)	Saturated fat (4 g) Moyad fat ratio 7:1 High in potassium (190 mg) High in selenium (6–8 times the RDA)
Cashews (160 calories)	High in monounsaturated fat (8 g) 3.3:1 Moyad fat ratio Potassium (160 mg)
Chestnuts (50–100 calories per 3 roasted nuts)	Equal amounts of monounsaturated (0.1 g), polyunsaturated (0.1 g) & saturated fat (0.1 g) Moyad fat ratio 2:1 Lowest in calories & fat & high in water content High in potassium (600 mg) & fiber (1.5 g) Only nut with vitamin C (about 10 mg)
Hazelnuts/filberts (180 calories)	High in monounsaturated fat (13 g) Moyad fat ratio 15:1 High in potassium (210 mg) & fiber (3 g)
Macadamia (200 calories)	Monounsaturated fat (17g) Polyunsaturated fat (0 g) Moyad fat ratio 5.5:1
Peanuts (170 calories)	Higher in monounsaturated (7 g) compared to polyunsaturated fat (4 g) Moyad fat ratio 5.5:1 High in potassium (190 mg) High in resveratrol (anti-aging compound?)
Pecans (200 calories)	High in monounsaturated fat (12 g) Moyad fat ratio 9:1 High in fiber (3 g)
Pine nuts (190 calories)	High in polyunsaturated fat (10g) Moyad fat ratio 15:1 High in potassium (170 mg)
Pistachios (160 calories)	High in monounsaturated fat (7 g) Moyad fat ratio 5.5:1 High in potassium (300 mg) & fiber (3 g)

Sesame seeds (200 calories)	Almost equal amounts of monounsaturated & polyunsaturated fats Moyad fat ratio 6:1 High in healthy plant estrogen High in calcium (350 mg), iron (5 mg), magnesium (125 mg), potassium (170 mg) & fiber (4 g)
Soy nuts (150 calories)	High in polyunsaturated fat (2 times more) compared to monounsaturated fat Moyad fat ratio 6 to 8:1 High in potassium (325 mg) & fiber (4 g)
Sunflower seeds (170 calories)	High in polyunsaturated fat (9g) Moyad fat ratio 12:1 High in potassium (240 mg) & fiber (3 g)
Walnuts (190 calories)	Highest omega-3 polyunsaturated fat (13 g) Highest nut source of plant omega-3 (ALA) Moyad fat ratio 8:1

Your Goal: Consume a variety of nuts and seeds in small to moderate amounts regularly to increase your intake of healthy nutrients and to reduce your intake of calories.

Step 20 around the B.S.—Oils, Oils, Oils

Please make sure you enjoy and take advantage of frequent cooking oil changes! Never be B.S.ed into believing that olive oil is the healthiest type of oil, because this is all marketing spin! Do not forget the Moyad ratio here, and you will soon realize that, as with fruits and vegetables and nuts, there is a variety of heart-healthy oils. And always watch those calories (120 calories per tablespoon unless you use them as cooking sprays).

Cooking oils that are high in monounsaturated fat, high in natural vitamin E, high in omega-3 fatty acids, and lower in saturated and trans fat are not only heart healthy but also seem to be all-body healthy. Oils such as soybean, canola, olive, and safflower are just some of the healthy oils out there. Utilize a variety of heart-healthy oils in moderation.

Dr. Moyad, why should I be as excited about other healthy oils, like canola oil and a variety of plant-based oils, because B.S. experts for years have been telling me that olive oil is the healthiest oil?

Get ready for a reality check! The FDA has authorized a qualified health claim for canola oil that it reduces the risk of coronary heart disease (CHD). Just when some people began to think that olive oil was the only healthy oil, several positive studies and an appeal to the FDA have now placed canola oil into an interesting health area.

The claim now allowed by the FDA on canola oil labels is the following: "Limited and not conclusive scientific evidence suggests that eating about one and a half (1.5) tablespoons (about 19 grams) of canola oil daily may reduce the risk of coronary heart disease due to the unsaturated fat content in canola oil. To achieve this possible benefit, canola oil is to replace a similar amount of saturated fat and not increase the total number of calories you eat in a day. One serving of this product contains [x] grams of canola oil."

Canola oil is unusually high (93 percent of its fat content) in healthy unsaturated fat, does not have cholesterol and trans fat, and is one of the lowest oils in terms of saturated fat (only 7 percent). This may cause a reduction in total blood cholesterol and reduce "bad cholesterol" or low-density lipoprotein (LDL). Canola oil also has a high heat tolerance, neutral taste, and a light, smooth texture. It can be used as a salad or vegetable oil, and it is common to blend this oil with other vegetable oils to produce items such as margarine, shortening, salad oil, and cooking oil.

Canola oil was originally processed from rapeseed, which is actually a toxic plant. In its original form it is an excellent insect repellant. However, the makers of canola oil point out that the toxic qualities of the original plant have been virtually eliminated in the final product. The FDA certified canola oil on January 28, 1985, as safe or generally recognized as safe (GRAS) for food use, as long as it contains no more than 2 percent erucic acid. Earlier, the American Soybean Association had opposed the name but later supported the name "canola oil" when Canada did lower the erucic acid content of the oil also sold in Canada. The battle for your attention when it comes to cooking oils or any healthy product is simply fierce!

In the past, the oil was 30–60 percent erucic acid, which is the most toxic substance, but canola oil today only carries between 0.3 and 1.2 percent, with an overall average of 0.6 percent. The plant is now genetically engineered in Canada from the rapeseed plant, which is a part of the mustard family of plants. For those of you who are wondering, canola is not the name of a natural plant, but a created or made-up word from the words *Canada* and *oil*. The name came from the Canadian government.

What about corn oil? Other oils ...?

The FDA has also decided to let corn oil products make a limited health advertisement claim for a heart benefit to consumers.

So, now let's play my favorite game, which is called "Dr. Moyad is president of the cooking oil association and needs to increase sales in this entire health category." You've never heard of this game? I am going to quickly show you why *using a diversity of plant-based oils makes more sense in moderation for your health compared to using only olive oil!*

Healthy Cooking Oils (Tablespoon of oil)	Moyad Fat Ratio & Nutrition
Almond oil (120 calories)	Moyad fat ratio 14:1
Apricot kernel oil (120 calories)	Moyad fat ratio 14:1
Avocado oil (120 calories)	Moyad fat ratio 7:1
Canola oil (120 calories)	Moyad fat ratio 13:1 Smoke point of 400 degrees!

Healthy Cooking Oils (Tablespoon of oil)	Moyad Fat Ratio & Nutrition
Coconut oil (120 calories)	Moyad fat ratio 1:6
Corn oil (120 calories)	Moyad fat ratio 6:1
Cottonseed oil (120 calories)	Moyad fat ratio 3:1
Flaxseed oil (130 calories)	Moyad fat ratio 8.5:1 (8 g of omega-3 or ALA, 2 g of omega-6 or linoleic acid & 3 g of oleic acid/ monounsaturated fat)
Grapeseed oil (120 calories)	Moyad fat ratio 13:1 Smoke point of 400 degrees!
Hazelnut oil (120 calories)	Moyad fat ratio 13:1
Macadamia nut oil (120 calories)	Moyad fat ratio 6:1 Smoke point of 410 degrees!
Olive oil (120 calories)	Moyad fat ratio 6:1
Palm oil (120 calories)	Moyad fat ratio 1:1
Peanut oil (120 calories)	Moyad fat ratio 3.5:1
Safflower oil (120 calories)	Moyad fat ratio 13:1 High in natural vitamin E
Sesame oil (120 calories)	Moyad fat ratio 6:1
Soybean oil (120 calories)	Moyad fat ratio 6:1
Sunflower oil (120 calories)	Moyad fat ratio 8.5:1
Walnut oil (120 calories)	Moyad fat ratio 6:1

Cooking oils with some of the highest monounsaturated fat levels include:

Macadamia nut oil (12 g)
Hazelnut oil (11 g)
Olive oil (11 g)
Safflower oil(10 g)
Almond oil (10 g)
Apricot kernel oil (10 g)
Avocado oil (10 g)

Cooking/plant oils with the most plant omega-3 fats include flaxseed oil, canola oil, walnut oil, and soybean oil. The oils lowest in saturated fat include canola oil, apricot kernel oil, safflower oil, hazelnut oil, almond oil, and grapeseed oil.

Your Goal: Look for a variety of heart-healthy and plant-based cooking oils to include in your diet.

**Please remember: Heart Healthy = All Healthy
and Heart Unhealthy = All Unhealthy!**

Step 21 around the B.S.—Plant Estrogens

Soy and flaxseed are some of the best sources for plant estrogens, but there are many other new sources being discovered that you should know about, such as sesame seeds. Getting these plant estrogens is another way to become more healthy.

| Dr. B.S.

"Soy products are the best source of plant estrogen, and they reduce the risk of breast and prostate cancer!"

| Dr. Moyad's No B.S.

"Whatever! Most healthy foods and beverages have some plant estrogens, but flaxseed and sesame seed have as much plant estrogen as soy. These foods are not only high in plant estrogen but soluble and insoluble fiber, and omega-3 fatty acids in the case of flaxseed, which makes them heart healthy."

The so-called plant estrogens are found in higher concentrations in soy, flaxseed, and now sesame seed products (seed, oil, powder). All of these products are heart healthy and may reduce your cholesterol. In addition, they are low in saturated and trans fats, higher in fiber, and are just overall healthy. The Food and Drug Administration (FDA) suggests that 25 grams a day of soy protein from a variety of traditional sources (soybeans, tofu, soy protein powder, soy milk) may reduce the risk of heart disease along with a reduction in saturated fat intake.

Review of Some of the Healthiest and Cheapest Traditional Soy Products
Listed by isoflavone (plant estrogen) and protein content with little to no saturated or trans fat

Soy Product	1 Serving	Total Isoflavones
Soybean	1/2 cup	175–200 mg
Tempeh	4 ounces	60 mg
Soy protein powder	1/3 cup	45 mg
Tofu	4 ounces	40 mg

Soy milk	1 cup	20 mg
Soy sauce*	10 gallons	0 mg

*Note: Soy sauce is listed for comparison purposes and not intended as a recommendation unless you catch a very large fish that requires larger than normal amounts of this sauce on your sushi. Also, if you are wise, you will choose the low-sodium soy sauce because it tastes the same but will not contribute as much to your high blood pressure.

Uncooked soy protein (only 2 servings a day) like that found in edamame, soy milk, soy nuts, soy powder, or tofu may lower LDL cholesterol by 8–10 percent. It seems that cooked soy protein like that in muffins or nutritional bars may not provide a benefit. Soy pills and protein bars are not that exciting. This is because they are, in general, expensive, unproven, and, in the case of the bars, generally loaded with calories and low in fiber.

Soy is big business and nutrition is big business, which means there are always forces out there trying to convince you that soy or its competitor (milk) comes with a catch. Having a serving or two of soy every day or on a regular basis is healthy and not associated with problems (except that some people have a soy allergy!). If you are willing to ingest megadoses of soy every day, then, as with everything else in this world, you will see a catch/side effect. In addition, it does not make much sense to go above moderation with soy because there are plenty of other great tasting and healthy foods that should get your attention, such as flaxseed powder!

Great Qualities of Ground Flaxseed

- Fiber (Ground regular brown flaxseed has a lot of fiber, but golden flaxseed has almost twice the fiber of regular flaxseed.)
- It has as much plant estrogen as soy (great for hot flash reduction) and about 250 mg of plant estrogens in 1–2 tablespoons).
- One of the largest sources of plant omega-3 fatty acids (1–2 tablespoons can provide as much as 1,500 to 2,000 mg of omega-3).
- It is one of the least expensive sources of flaxseed (costs pennies a day).
- It is the form of flaxseed that has gone through the largest number of successful human clinical trials (including a recent

clinical study for hot flash reduction and possible prostate cancer prevention).
- It is very low in calories!
- It actually has a neutral or nutty taste, so you will just like it!

Where do I purchase flaxseed?

Whole and ground flaxseed may be purchased in the vitamin/supplement department of most retailers carrying these types of products.

How do I grind the flaxseed?

You can grind it in a coffee grinder or even a cheap spice grinder, but today you don't have to do this task. There are plenty of companies that offer vacuum-packed or canned or sealed containers of ground flaxseed. I purchase these products because I am not patient enough every day to grind the flaxseed! Are you? Please do not answer this question until you have tried to grind it up yourself for thirty straight days.

What is the difference between golden flaxseed and regular brown flaxseed?

Golden flaxseed is usually a little more expensive and contains more fiber—as much as twice the regular form of flaxseed. So, if you want to increase your fiber intake, golden flaxseed is a good choice, but you cannot go wrong with either form of flaxseed.

What are the side effects of flaxseed?

Just as with any other strong source of fiber, if you get too much (more than a few tablespoons a day) you will have one big advantage over anyone else in that you will get more reading done (reading *War and Peace* twice should be no problem).

I am not a big fan of most flaxseed dietary supplements because they are generally expensive, have very limited research, and have no fiber. Flaxseed oil is not cheap, needs refrigeration, expires after a while, has questionable taste, and has *no fiber*. However, used on salads it is a way to get your plant estrogens and omega-3 daily intake. It also has about 120 to 130 calories per tablespoon, so you are not going to lose weight in general on the flaxseed oil diet. It is healthy to eat flaxseeds whole, but you will not absorb as much omega-3 fatty acid or plant estrogen nor enjoy the full fiber benefit. Flaxseed meal (pre-ground) is also healthy, but check for the fiber content.

What about breast cancer and plant estrogens?

I think the evidence is good that these plant estrogens from soy, flaxseed, and sesame seed may *reduce the risk of bone loss, breast cancer, and prostate cancer.* If you have been treated for breast cancer, the general consensus is that you stay away from soy, flaxseed, and sesame seed because they contain the highest quantities of "plant estrogen." But the amount of plant estrogens is really so low and the concentration so weak that it rarely changes estrogen levels unless you eat mega-quantities daily. This is a better-safe-than-sorry recommendation.

In reality, I let patients make their own decision on this one. I tell them that we have no clarity on the issue, but I personally would not worry about this too much when such foods are consumed in moderation. Let's look at flaxseed as an example. Flaxseed is much more than plant estrogen, because it also has omega-3s, fiber, low calories, other healthy fats like oleic acid (like that found in olive oil), lowers cholesterol, and much more that we all agree are *healthy for breast cancer patients*! Breast cancer patients should do what they feel is most comfortable for them on this one. What do you do when there is no real good human research in this area? You state the facts, and your opinion, and you let people make the decision they feel is appropriate for them. Most estrogen-positive breast cancer patients, in my opinion, reduce their intake just to be safe, and most estrogen-negative patients seem to be split on this issue.

Recent research has also demonstrated that sesame seeds have as much plant estrogen as flaxseed and soy, but not as much fiber as flaxseed. It is also a wonderful natural source of vitamin E. So, for example, if I am going after hot flashes, I would use all or at least one of these natural products.

Your Goal: Consume more food sources of plant estrogens.

**Please remember: Heart Healthy = All Healthy
and Heart Unhealthy = All Unhealthy!**

Step 22 around the B.S.—Sex, Sleep, Smoking, Stress & Sodium

Get more sex and sleep now. (I inserted this in here so no one could say I did not talk about it in my book.) I will not say much more about this, because if you follow the rest of the steps you should sleep better. Little to no sleep = reduced immune health = heart unhealthy = all unhealthy = you probably are not getting much sex! Do not be afraid to get some temporary sleep assistance (from melatonin at 0.5 to 1 mg/day, to valerian from 400 to 600 mg/day as a dietary supplement, to the prescription meds).

Stop smoking now! If you smoke, do not be shy to try going "cold turkey" with your health-care professional pushing you to do so. By the way, in clinical research from the National Cancer Institute, cold turkey has been as successful as many of the antismoking methods, pills, patches, and gums. In addition, Chantix® (a new drug from Pfizer) looks to be an effective pill, but keep up to date with the ongoing safety of the product as it is still a big issue. Behavioral therapy should be combined with other methods. Perhaps the last resort of anti-smoking success is using smokeless tobacco (no kidding) in small pouches to continue to get a nicotine rush that you can adjust until you are able to finally quit! Overall, it is the lesser of two evils, and the end will justify the means! (How many B.S. experts are freaking out right now?! Well, bring it on!)

Lower your mental and physical stress now. More stress = reduced immune health = heart unhealthy = all unhealthy. Stress reduction through many methods, such as music, controlled breathing, support groups, yoga, golf ... has been shown to reduce blood pressure as much as 5 to 10 points.

Reduce your sodium intake now! (This is critical.) Become more aware of sodium right now, but not necessarily by removing the saltshaker. The relation between more sodium and higher blood pressure is as clear as the visible bumps and lumps seen in the middle-age man wearing one of those antiquated really tight and tiny swimsuits at the local pool. (Okay, I also had to wear one of those as a kid, which is why I had no friends ... thanks a lot, Mom and Dad.) Compare similar beverages and foods, and choose the one that is lower in sodium. Feel free to use a salt substitute (potassium chloride, for example), more spices, low amounts of more flavorful sea salt. ... Keep in mind that the number-one cause of death for over 100 years has been cardiovascular disease, but the number-one cause of cardiovascular death around the world right now is actually high blood pressure! Ouch!

| Dr. B.S.

"Sodium is a problem, so you need to remove your saltshaker now!"

| Dr. Moyad's No B.S.

"Whatever! Sodium in the saltshaker is a minor issue! So it is okay to still shake, shake, shake, shake, shake, shake, shake your saltshaker. (I think this comes from KC & the Sunshine Band, circa 1970s ... oops, no, that was shake your booty not your saltshaker.) Processed foods contain about 80 percent of the excess sodium that we consume, so the smartest thing you can do is to simply begin to compare beverage and food labels!"

"Anything with sodium in it."—Coach Bill Belichick of the New England Patriots and the coach of Tom Brady, the greatest quarterback ever ... when the coach was asked by the media what his secret daily diet is, because he is one of the most famous coaching minds of all time, except when that perfect season was ruined by the Giants—hey, maybe it was the sodium that gave him high blood pressure and did not allow him to think clearly that day?

Let's clear the air quickly on the sodium subject. One of the largest government-funded studies in the history of medicine that you, the taxpayer, paid for was called the DASH (Dietary Approaches to Stop Hypertension) study. The great thing about this original study was that it involved pre-hypertensive people not taking prescription medications. Half of the participants were women, and 60 percent were African-Americans, and this also made the study remarkable. Fast forward several years, and it was amazing to find out what a wonderful impact eating healthy and lowering sodium intake had on blood pressure numbers. Let me first show you below how incredible the findings were with the DASH diet compared to our most commonly sold prescription medications.

Currently, the healthy recommendation is to get 2,300 milligrams of sodium (1 teaspoon) per day, but in the DASH diet the effective dose was 1,500 milligrams (less than a teaspoon) of sodium per day. Most people are consuming 3,500 to 4,500 milligrams per day!

So, see the table for how diet and salt reduction are just as beneficial as any blood pressure–lowering drug therapy. Imagine what would happen if you added exercise, weight loss, and alcohol reduction.

Effects of Treatment on Blood Pressure

Blood Pressure Lowering Treatment Class or Therapy	Reduction in Blood Pressure
DASH diet + maximum of 1,500 mg of salt/day (less than a teaspoon)	Systolic = –11 mmHg Diastolic = –6 mmHg
ACE (angiotensin-converting enzyme) inhibitor drug such as captopril (e.g., Capoten®)	Systolic = –6 mmHg Diastolic = –5 mmHg
Alpha-blocker such as prazosin (e.g., Minipress®)	Systolic = –9 mmHg Diastolic = –6 mmHg
Beta-blocker such as atenolol (e.g., Tenormin®)	Systolic = –8 mmHg Diastolic = –7 mmHg
Calcium channel blocker such as diltiazem (e.g., Cardizem®)	Systolic = –10 mmHg Diastolic = –9 mmHg
Thiazide diuretic such as hydrochlorothiazide	Systolic = –11 mmHg Diastolic = –5 mmHg

Keep in mind that about 80 percent of your daily sodium comes from food processing and only about 5 percent from the saltshaker (5 percent in cooking and 10 percent occurs naturally). So, let's look at the sodium ranges of some common beverages and foods, and you'll see why *comparing labels is so powerful.*

- Breads = 100–200 mg of sodium in 1 ounce.
- Chicken with rice soup (condensed) = 600–1,300 mg in ½ a cup.
- Frozen pizza (plain) = 400–1,200 mg of sodium in 4 ounces.
- Frozen vegetables = 5–150 mg of sodium in ½ a cup.
- Potato chips = 100 to 200 mg of sodium in 1 ounce.
- Pretzels = 250 to 600 mg of sodium in 1 ounce.
- Salad dressing (regular) = 50 to 250 mg of sodium in 1 tablespoon.
- Salsa = 75 to 150 mg of sodium in 1 tablespoon.
- Tomato juice = 350 to 1,000 mg of sodium in 8 ounces.
- Tomato soup = 600 to 1,300 mg of sodium in ½ cup.

Whether a person has high blood pressure or not, and whether she/he is on a blood pressure medication or not, the message is very clear. Moderately changing diet to reduce blood pressure works and includes the following Moyad-modified DASH diet changes:

Specific DASH Study Dietary Recommendations to Reduce Blood Pressure	Easier-to-Follow Dr. Moyad Translation
Fats and oils (2–3 servings/day, or 27% of calories from fat)	"Choose healthy plant-based fats (monounsaturated & polyunsaturated) over less healthy fats." (1 tablespoon = 120 calories, so use cooking sprays when possible)
Fruits and vegetables (4–5 servings of *each* per day)	"Get more fiber, magnesium & potassium from a diversity of real fruits & vegetables."
Grains (7–8 servings/day)	"Get more fiber from products such as whole wheat pasta or bread & pick the one with lower sodium amounts!"
Low-fat or fat-free dairy (2–3 servings/day)	"Get more calcium & protein from food and choose healthy fats over less healthy fats."
Meats, poultry & fish (2 or less servings/day)	"Get more magnesium, omega-3 oils & protein from food. Choose lean meats, trim away visible fat, and bake, boil, broil, or roast rather than fry. Occasionally OK to eat the skin." (Serving size = deck of cards.)
Nuts, seeds & dry beans (4–5 servings/week)	"Get more fiber, magnesium, potassium & healthy fats from foods." (Serving size = a handful.)
Sodium (1,500 mg or less/day)	"Try not to specifically measure your sodium intake. Instead, when buying canned or frozen vegetables, select those with no salt added or low salt; use fresh fish, lean meat & poultry rather than canned or processed food; use herbs, salt-free/Lite/substitute, or sea salt or spices in cooking."

Specific DASH Study Dietary Recommendations to Reduce Blood Pressure	Easier-to-Follow Dr. Moyad Translation
Sweets (5/week)	"Eat more low-calorie foods and limit your intake of high-calorie fast foods and sweets."

Note: There is a difference between salt (sodium chloride) and sodium. If you really want to know, there are 400 milligrams of sodium in 1 gram of salt or sodium chloride. Remember, it is the sodium level with which we are concerned, and that is what has to be reported on labels.

Your Goal: Reduce your sodium intake.

**Please remember: Heart Healthy = All Healthy
and Heart Unhealthy = All Unhealthy!**

Step 23 around the B.S.—The Final Step & Now the Smell Should Be Almost Gone!

Moderation is the key to life, and humans were not meant to abuse their machines/bodies, nor were they meant to have an unhealthy obsession with health. Focus on the forest over the tree(s) as much as possible when it comes to your health and any future diet or lifestyle-changing advice or program. When Dr. B.S. recommends something specific, ask yourself what the greater general message is within the recommendation. For example, when someone says pomegranate, think about a variety of fruits and vegetables that you like to eat; when someone says olive oil, think about a variety of healthy plant oils that you like; when someone says salmon, think about a variety of fish high in omega-3s that you like to eat; when someone says Brazil nuts, think about a variety of healthy nuts and seeds you like to consume; when someone says you should only be jogging, think about a variety of exercises that make you feel good; when someone says use only free weights to build muscle, think of any of situation that gives you resistance exercise from stretchable bands to Nautilus to push-ups.

| Dr. B.S.

"Just get more _____ (insert a ridiculous or naïve prevention tip), and you can become healthier overnight!"

| Dr. Moyad's No B.S.

"Whatever! The more you can do in moderation the bigger the payoff! I would rather have a patient who can do multiple things in moderation compared to one or two healthy things in excess."

When it comes to fad diets, what should I do?

First, try to understand some of the behaviors involved with these diets, their advantages and disadvantages, and which diet or program *fits your personality*. All of them have inherent positives and negatives.

Talk to your doctor or a nutritionist about these diets, but most depend on lowering your intake of calories and exercising more. Regardless, the primary goal is to maintain a healthy weight/cholesterol/blood pressure, and one diet or program does not necessarily work for everyone. I am a fan of programs like Weight Watchers®, for example, because they teach you about food, moderation, and portion sizes, and are motivating because they also involve working with a support group. Also, they are backed by not only personal testimony but also actual clinical research. Low-carbohydrate diets may work for many individuals, but long-term they can be a challenge. Regardless of what you choose, I am a big fan of risk assessment, education, and picking a comprehensive or forest-over-the-tree program that is *moderate, practical, and realistic*!

One of the most famous studies that you, the taxpayer, paid for was conducted by the National Cancer Institute and involved about 380,000 men and women. It showed a reduction in not just cardiovascular disease but certain cancers. This pattern has also been associated with lower risks of eye diseases and many other conditions like Alzheimer's disease, for example, obtainable by following a Mediterranean pattern diet. In the following table, participants received 1 point for each dietary change, and the more points, the lower the risk. Individuals with scores above 6 began to see a significantly lower risk of dying over the next 10 years from heart disease or cancer compared with those who had a score less than 4. The lesson here is as clear as the forest—the more you can do in moderation, the better your odds of living longer and better. So, what is your score?

Beverage/Food & Other Comments about the Mediterranean Pattern	Circle Yes or No Each time you answer "yes," give yourself one point.
Alcohol average intake of 1/2 to 1 drink for women & 1 to 2 drinks a day for men	Yes No (Notice I did not specify which type of alcohol is the best for your health.)
Fat intake focused on healthy fats that have mostly monounsaturated or polyunsaturated fat (canola, olive, safflower oil …) compared to saturated fat	Yes No (Notice I did not specify which oil is the best for your health.)
Fish intake of 4 or more servings per week	Yes No (Notice I did not specify which fish is best for your health.)

Fruit intake of 3 or more servings a day	Yes No (Notice I did not specify which fruit is best for your health.)
Legumes/beans intake of 2 or more servings per week	Yes No (Notice I did not specify which legumes/beans are the best for your health.)
Meat intake of less than 2 servings a day (especially red and processed meat)	Yes No (Notice how some regular consumption of meat is allowed if you want to eat it.)
Nuts & seed intake of 2 or more servings a week	Yes No (Notice I did not specify which nuts or seeds are the best for your health.)
Vegetables (other than potatoes) intake of 4 or more servings a day	Yes No (Notice I did not specify which vegetable is best for your health.)
Whole grain intake of 2 or more servings a day (only whole grain versions of bagel, cereal, bread, bun, muffin, pasta, rice ...)	Yes No (Notice I did not specify which whole grains are the best for your health & I guess eating bread & pasta is okay for you.)
Total score	Points _____

Note: Traditional Mediterranean diets also allow moderate intake of dairy such as cheese, milk, and yogurt.

Personally, I like the Mediterranean diet because it is a real moderate and diverse diet with many components. Basically, this is an "everything in moderation" diet. Work with your health professional to find a diet or dietary program that makes sense for you. Your health professional should monitor your major numbers such as cholesterol, blood pressure, weight loss, and other risk assessment numbers while on a new type of diet to make sure it is working for you.

What is the difference between a ketogenic low-carbohydrate diet and a non-ketogenic low-carbohydrate diet?

Low-carbohydrate diets come in two forms:

1. Ketogenic low-carbohydrate ("Atkins"-type) diets usually involve starting out by eating very small amounts of complex and simple carbohydrates (less than 20 grams of net carbs per day) and are essentially very high in fat (60 percent of caloric intake, and 20 percent of this is saturated), but include more monounsaturated and polyunsaturated fat, more cholesterol, and less fiber.

2. Non-ketogenic low-carbohydrate diets ("lower-fat" or "zone-type diet") usually involve more than 20–40 grams of net carbs per day and are lower in fat (30 percent of caloric intake and less than 10 percent from saturated fat), lower in cholesterol, higher in fiber, and higher in low-fat meats and low-fat dairy products; and they allow more fruits and vegetables.

Both types of low-carbohydrate diets can help you lose weight *equally*, but some research has shown that the non-ketogenic type of diet seems to give better emotional well-being while you are dieting. Talk to your doctor about which diet is appropriate for you if you want to go low-carb.

You should also keep in mind one very important thing about lifestyle changes and diet. Today, more than ever before, it seems that individuals are inundated with lots of small changes about diet that apparently make a difference. For example, there is a lot of attention given in the media about things such as organic versus inorganic fruits and vegetables, artificial sweeteners, caffeine, sugar, chocolate, and other changes that apparently make a difference. However, does reducing your intake of these things really make a difference? I do not think so, and even if they did, these changes take the focus off the bigger changes that may truly make a difference.

You see, it is easy to have an unhealthy obsession with health in today's world. The major changes should really get all the attention, but in reality they receive little attention. Weight loss, exercise, a moderate healthy diet, reducing blood pressure and cholesterol—these should be receiving the attention. Instead, focusing on your caffeine intake is okay, but only after you take care of the forest before the tree. The next time your attention is diverted to things such as coffee and artificial sweeteners, remember to shift your focus back to cholesterol, blood pressure, weight maintenance, exercise, and other essential items, because these can really make a difference. We should move toward better health one No B.S. step at a time. Looking back on these steps as a whole, you can see the sheer power they have on our lives!

So, I will leave you with the most important part of the book—a modified version of the 52 countries study, which was completed in, you guessed it, 52 countries and found that we are different in terms only of where we live, and that when it comes to health advice we are, in general, the exact same. Regardless of age, color, race, creed, gender, or genetics, the more you were able to do in moderation the bigger the potential payoff in terms of probability. Rate yourself in the following table, which is a partial Dr. Moyad summary of the moderate lifestyle changes that in combination may reduce the risk of a first cardiovascular event and of dying young by approximately 85–95 percent (according to a combination of lifestyle studies including the 52 countries study, Honolulu Heart Study , and others). Note that each healthy change was associated with an approximately 5–10 percent reduction!

Moyad Moderate Lifestyle Changes	Yes (Each "yes" is a 5–10% improvement in your health or a 5–10% reduction in your risk.)	No (Keep in mind that if you are being treated for any of these 10 conditions and they are now normal due to treatment, well, you should count this as a "yes" in my opinion.)
1. Do you consume alcohol in moderation (at least once a week but not more than 1–2 servings per day)?		
2. Do you have low to normal blood pressure? (Not even pre-hypertension is allowed here.)		

Moyad Moderate Lifestyle Changes	Yes (Each "yes" is a 5–10% improvement in your health or a 5–10% reduction in your risk.)	No (Keep in mind that if you are being treated for any of these 10 conditions and they are now normal due to treatment, well, you should count this as a "yes" in my opinion.)
3. Do you have fantastic cholesterol numbers (low LDL & triglycerides & high HDL or a low Apo B to Apo A ratio)? (see Step 1, Fasting Cholesterol Test)		
4. Are you free of any major mental stress or depression?		
5. Do you consume fruits & vegetables more than just one time a day?		
6. Do you have low to normal glucose blood levels?		
7. Are you a non-smoker?		
8. Do you do at least 30–45 minutes a day of moderate physical activity/exercise on average (4 or more hours a week)?		

9. Do you have a normal waist circumference (WC) or a normal waist-to-hip ratio (WHR)?		
10. Do you lift weights or do some resistance exercise several times a week?		
Bonus for men only: Are you married? (Only men had a health benefit, no kidding. Did women have a health benefit being married? Well, let's just say I do not talk about this study with my wife.)		
Total number of "yes" & "no" answers		

Keep in mind that there was about a 70 percent chance of living to age 85 if individuals had all or most of the ten healthy factors at midlife observed by the researchers, and a 55 percent chance of being in the "exceptional survival" group, which means they lived to be at least 85 years old and were in amazing health with no signs of physical or mental disease or disability, including *not* having specific conditions including cancer (except non-melanoma skin cancer), diabetes, heart disease, lung disease (chronic obstructive pulmonary disease or COPD), Parkinson's disease, or stroke.

However, there was only a 22 percent chance of living to age 85 years (with disease or disability) if in midlife the individual had three or fewer of the healthy practices, and less than a 10 percent chance of being in the "exceptional survival" group.

Let's play pretend … If the ten healthy factors were discussed as if they were a pill discovered by me, and the public could take this pill daily for these overall benefits, this study would have made the cover of every major newspaper in the world, and I would have been given a Nobel Prize ASAP! However, it is only a lifestyle study! It is not sexy enough for a Nobel Prize for the researchers that started and completed it, but those people deserve it. In other words, just because this is a lifestyle study and not a pill or medical intervention study, *I believe most individuals will never hear that it was published or even what it means unless the readers of this book do something about it and teach others about it (yes, including your children).*

Your Goal: Live a life of moderation while making healthy lifestyle changes.

In case you forgot, **Heart Healthy = All Healthy,
and Heart Unhealthy = All Unhealthy!**

Part IV

Dr. Moyad's No B.S. Practical, Realistic & Probability-Based Pill Suggestions

| Dr. B.S. or a B.S. Commercial

"Nutraceuticals or nutrition supplement companies are evil ... and pharmaceutical companies are evil!"

| Dr. Moyad's No B.S.

"Whatever!" It is unrealistic to identify some terrible generalized enemy and ask you to support one side only. This is similar to someone telling me I have to be a Democrat or Republican and follow everything they feel and believe. We have great nutritional and pharmaceutical companies, and we have some really terrible nutritional and pharmaceutical companies. These companies are simply a microcosm of society itself."

The public and health-care professionals need to stay consistent because otherwise there would be chaos in medicine. What do I mean by this statement? We have come to rely on pharmaceutical drugs having a certain amount of beneficial evidence to support their use before a doctor recommends them and patients request them. However, somewhere things have gotten a little out of hand. We have allowed the dollar and almost a type of below-the-radar bullying by certain aggressive companies to change the way some of us indirectly or directly think and how we recommend products.

Look, I am also guilty here of at times making the problem a little worse, but I have learned over time what it should take to recommend any pill. I began to seek companies (nutritional or pharmaceutical) that were healthy. My job is to be an objective educator about conventional and alternative options. In other words, the drugs/supplements that meet the following criteria are the ones that in my opinion should be recommended the most by health-care professionals for the public and simply utilized the most *when the first part of this book cannot take care of the issue or problem.* So, a pill company should at least meet these ten criteria.

How to Evaluate a Pill

1. Is its use supported by published human research and not just test-tube or animal research?

What this means is that if I had a dime for every pill that worked in the laboratory but did not work at all in humans, well, I would be rich! Of course, laboratory research is impressive, but do not let that determine what pill you should take. Unfortunately, that is what is happening right now with many dietary supplements. Hey, if you are a test tube or mouse, we can cure you of any disease right now! Otherwise, there should be research with people and the results should have been published in a reputable medical journal, presenting them for objective peer review and criticism. Oh, and if you do not have any research, do not B.S. the public and say that you do!

2. Has the company shown financial dedication and real commitment to ongoing research?

Do you ever notice that the greatest thing about a company or pill that has *no research* is that it has *no research*? In other words, these companies and their experts are the greatest Monday morning quarterbacks in the business. Whether it's natural hormone replacement versus synthetic or calcium carbonate versus calcium citrate supplements, these people will twist, manipulate, and criticize someone else's research but fail to mention that their product has undergone absolutely no long-term credible research. The companies that commit to ongoing research simply should get your attention and commitment.

You cannot have research without some serious financial investment. I hear from so many dietary supplement and pharmaceutical companies that claim that they are mom-and-pop and so small that they cannot compete with the bigger companies, so they cannot invest in research, but their product is great. I don't see it that way. I see mom-and-pop companies doing things the right way almost every day. Nothing in life and medicine in general comes easy without some serious time and money invested. I am all in favor of companies and researchers making a fortune after they have spent time proving that their product for your health is truly better. Also, a long-term commitment to research makes me more likely to commit long-term to a company.

3. What is the level of effectiveness, and who should and should not use the product?

After all the research and financial commitment, the company should be able to identify to some degree who does and does not benefit from the product and why. It is that simple. If you sell a vitamin or another pill, what type of person actually needs it based on your research or does *not* need it? If you say, or simply imply, that everyone needs this pill right now without focusing on the small print or who does not need your pill, then you are the King or Queen of B.S. This is the problem I am having right now with some (not all) of the commercials for aspirin, cholesterol remedies, cough suppressants for kids and adults, and many calcium and multivitamin commercials.

4. What about safety and quality control (is it at least heart healthy, mentally healthy and ideally healthy in pregnancy and this includes dietary supplements)?

The FDA has a new policy, with which I completely agree in this one area, and I think it is wonderful! If a product *is not heart healthy*, there is a good chance it will no longer be on the market or get approved for most conditions. Vioxx®, Zelnorm®, ephedra, and Torceptrapib are now gone, and now Avandia® is in trouble (great drugs/supplements but bad for the heart). Also, if a pill *is not mentally healthy*, why should you take it? Ideally, it is nice to know that the product is safe if taken during pregnancy. What this means is that *the benefit of taking the pill should always outweigh the risk of taking it.*

5. Is it affordable?

What is the company doing to make the product affordable? If the product is expensive, what is the company doing for the people who cannot afford it? I am not a big fan of giving what I call the "objective, financially dependent skewed consultation." In other words, I should be giving the same advice to the person in the mansion in Beverly Hills compared to the person in the lowest income bracket in the Los Angeles area.

6. What about compliance, formulations, and flexibility?

A medicine or pill can be the best in the world, but if a person does not find it easy to take, then he or she will not take it. Whether or not a pill is life-saving, research clearly shows that it is only taken on a regular basis by 50 percent of the people who are given it after just a few years. Anyone can take any pill for 3 months, but for 3 or 5 years—that is a completely different story. Companies need to help with ways to improve the ease of taking any pill by offering different formulations (spray, under the tongue, strip, pill …).

7–10. Is the company responsible?

Responsibility encompasses distribution of a company's knowledge and products to people regardless of background or financial status, and just doing the right damn thing.

I primarily work with companies that meet all ten Moyad criteria. These are healthy companies that realize that when you do the right thing it is great for the company, the patient, the health-care professional ... it is truly win-win-win! They are not shy about getting samples to the hard-hit hurricane areas of Louisiana or simply other areas in need. They are not focused on giving doctors gifts or fancy hotel rooms, but are focused on teaching them how to better serve their patients. These companies do not hesitate to provide a nutritional booklet, class, or tape measure for waist circumference measurements or in supporting the cancer patient groups—in other words, companies with a *certain sense of purpose beyond profit*. In other words, they carry a certain sense of *responsibility*.

The Most Important Pills to Discuss with Your Doctor (Prescriptions and Dietary Supplements)

Acid Reflux Over-the-Counter & Prescription Medications

| Dr. B.S.

"Acid reflux drugs are perfectly safe and do not come with side effects, and that is why they are some of the most widely prescribed medications in the world!"

| Dr. Moyad's No B.S.

"Whatever!" Acid in your stomach is necessary for better immune health. Acid reflux drugs are completely over-prescribed, and too many people are on these medications for too long a period of time!"

Stomach acid is good for you. Yes, it is the body's major protector against a variety of ugly bugs. Think about this for a second. If you swallow some ugly virus or bacteria that you cannot see and it hits the stomach where the acidity is enough to normally burn a hole in your carpet, what do you think is going to happen to that bug? BAM (I sound like that chef on TV.) Most of the time the bug will lose the fight.

Acid reflux medications work by reducing the amount of acid in your stomach, so why are acid reflux medications basically the number-one prescribed drugs in the world? This is because some people might make too much stomach acid and get heartburn, but when did heartburn become such a worldwide epidemic? For years, Dr. B.S.s claimed that these drugs are so safe that they do not come with side effects. Every effective drug, surgery, or even dietary supplement comes with a side effect or a catch. In the past few years, human studies have found that long-term use of acid reflux medications may slightly increase the risk of bone loss or osteoporosis (you will have trouble absorbing calcium), pneumonia, and serious infections in the gastrointestinal tract.

There is a minority of people who do not do well with any type of acid reflux because it can increase their risk of esophageal cancer. These individuals need to be on medication long-term, but again these folks should be the exception and not the rule.

It is not B.S. to tell you that these drugs are miracle drugs for the people who need them, but they are completely over-prescribed and used in patients for too long. Every person on these medications should reevaluate with their doctor every few months whether or not they should stay on these medications. In some patients, just losing a few pounds and increasing your fiber intake can reduce the amount of drug you need or eventually eliminate it entirely, which should be the ultimate goal. Another option is to reduce the amount of the drug and eventually switch to calcium carbonate supplements, because they not only help with the heartburn but can also reduce your risk of bone loss and numerous other health problems. (See calcium and vitamin D.)

Aspirin

| Dr. B.S.

"Everyone over the age of forty should take a daily aspirin. Aspirin can reduce your risk of a first heart attack and may reduce the risk of some cancers, so everyone should take it because it is a miracle drug, natural, and over the counter."

| Dr. Moyad's No B.S.

"Whatever! Aspirin is a miracle drug for the individuals who *qualify* for it, but it can be a potential disaster if you do not qualify for it and you are taking it right now! It should *not* be taken just to reduce your risk of some cancers, including colon cancer. It is completely ridiculous, reckless, and dangerous for any doctor or health-care professional to make blanket statements and simply recommend taking any pill daily, including aspirin, for men and women of a specific age without knowing if she or he actually qualifies for it. Just because you are a certain age does not mean that you qualify for it!"

Aspirin is a compound that was originally taken from willow bark. In the old days, people realized that if you chewed on willow bark it could reduce pain and discomfort caused by a number of conditions.

The sales and the popularity of aspirin really took off after a very famous study known as the Physicians Health Study (PHS) was published. This clinical trial only included male doctors. In the PHS, only healthy male physicians who took a regular-strength aspirin every other day experienced a 44 percent reduction in the risk of first heart attack. However, aspirin did *not* significantly reduce the risk of dying younger from all causes as some people believe, and it did not significantly reduce the risk of stroke. In addition, the incidence of bleeding complications was higher in the aspirin group compared to the placebo group. The benefit compared to the risk was only greater for those individuals who had a moderate to higher risk of having a first heart attack. This study demonstrated that aspirin is only a miracle drug for the people who need it, but a disaster for the people (men or women) who do not need it!

The FDA has *never* approved the use of aspirin to reduce the risk of a first heart attack in low to average heart-disease-risk individuals, because most people at low risk for a heart attack would have a greater risk of complications and potentially life-threatening side effects compared to benefits. Also, in individuals who do not have heart disease, aspirin seemed to reduce the risk of nonfatal heart attacks more than fatal heart attacks. It all comes down to risk-to-benefit ratio and working with your doctor to see if you qualify for a medication.

If you and your doctor determine that your Framingham risk score is much lower than 10 percent, then aspirin is probably not for you. If your risk of heart disease is close to 10–20 percent, then you may qualify for aspirin; and if your risk is high, then you are potentially a good candidate for aspirin. Regardless, keep in mind that *by stopping smoking and lowering your blood pressure and cholesterol, you can reduce your Framingham risk score.*

How do I really know if I am a candidate for aspirin?

The following table is a list of current expert groups or authors and what they recommend when it comes to taking aspirin for the prevention of a first heart attack.

Level of Risk Needed Before Qualifying to Take Aspirin for the Prevention of a First Heart Attack

Organization/Authors	10-Year Risk of Coronary Heart Disease
American Heart Association (AHA)	Greater than 10%
U.S. Preventive Services Task Force	Greater than 6%
Past analysis by a group of experts (2001)	Greater than 15%

Organization/Authors	10-Year Risk of Coronary Heart Disease
Recent re-analysis by a group of experts	Equal to or greater than 7.5%
Overall Combined Recommendation	Between 6 and 15% risk

Keep in mind that patients who qualify for aspirin therapy should have normal blood pressure, because having high blood pressure while on any blood-thinning pill can only increase your risk of internal bleeding. Doses of 75 to 81 mg a day may be better for reducing the risk of side effects of aspirin compared to a dose of 325 mg/day. In women, the safest and most effective dosage ever tested was 100 mg every other day. Baby aspirin works as well as regular aspirin in many situations, and immediate-release aspirin works a little better than enteric-coated, but some individuals need to take enteric-coated or have to take aspirin with an acid-suppressive drug to reduce their risk of ulcers.

In women, aspirin to prevent heart attacks and strokes plays out a little differently. The Women's Health Study (WHS) of almost 40,000 women was the best study yet to determine the impact of taking a baby aspirin (actually 100 mg/day) every other day in healthy and generally middle-aged women for ten years. Women reduced their risk of a heart attack and stroke if they were at high risk (generally older than 65 years), but overall middle-aged or younger women did not benefit from aspirin, and aspirin did not significantly reduce the risk of cancer, including breast and colon cancer. Aspirin did *not* significantly reduce the risk of dying younger from any cause.

Long-term daily aspirin use can significantly increase your risk of hemorrhagic stroke (bleeding into the brain and other areas), gastrointestinal bleeding, gastrointestinal bleeding serious enough to require a blood transfusion, peptic ulcer, blood in the urine, easy bruising, and nosebleeds.

In men, aspirin reduces the risk of heart attack better than reducing the risk of strokes. Therefore, men at a high risk for a first heart attack should consider taking aspirin after a discussion with their doctor. In women the opposite finding has occurred (aspirin reduces ischemic stroke better than heart attack), so women should consider taking aspirin if there is a high risk for an ischemic stroke (type of stroke that occurs from a blockage in the arteries).

There are more than 15,000 deaths and more than 100,000 hospital admissions a year in the United States alone due to aspirin and non-steroidal anti-inflammatory drug pain relievers. Keep that in mind the next time you decide you want to pop aspirin daily like a vitamin without talking to your doctor first.

Blood Pressure–Reducing Drugs, Supplements, and Diets

| Dr. B.S.

"Diet and exercise do not work as well as a drug for blood pressure reduction!"

| Dr. Moyad's No B.S.

"Whatever! High blood pressure is the number-one cause of cardio-vascular disease deaths around the world, and high blood pressure simply destroys everything in its path, including the heart, kidneys, and sexual organs. So, blood pressure–lowering drugs are great, and diet and exercise improve the effect of the blood pressure drugs and may even help some patients to reduce the drug dosage or eliminate it entirely."

First, let's briefly discuss blood pressure drugs.

Blood Pressure Drug*	How It Works
ACE (angiotensin-converting enzyme) inhibitors and ARBs (angiotensin II receptor blockers)	Work to relax and increase or widen the size of the blood vessels. (ACE inhibitors can cause a nonserious but annoying dry cough; ARBs do not have this issue.)
Beta-blockers	Block a hormone that can cause multiple cardiac problems and can also slow the heart rate. (Can cause fatigue/lack of energy.)
Calcium channel blockers	Work to relax and increase or widen the size of the blood vessels. (Can cause ankle swelling.)

Blood Pressure Drug*	How It Works
Diuretics	Flush excess water and sodium from the body. (You can become dehydrated and lose electrolytes, especially potassium.)

*These drugs can be used in combination, or by themselves, but regardless of how used they are miracle drugs for the individuals that need them. Always look for generic and cheaper versions of these drugs.

It is also amazing that lifestyle changes also have such a large impact on blood pressure. Let's look at some basic lifestyle changes and how they can affect blood pressure in less than a few months. All of these changes may be combined with or used without drug therapy.

Lifestyle Changes That Are Moderate, Practical & Realistic	Average Reduction in Systolic Blood Pressure	Average Reduction in Diastolic Blood Pressure
Alcohol intake reduced to moderation, periodic intake, or eliminated	−4 mmHg	−2 to −3 mmHg
Dietary changes in moderation with salt/sodium restriction (beans, chicken, fish, fruits & vegetables, lean meat, low-fat dairy, nuts, seeds, whole grains)	−11 mmHg	−5 to −6 mmHg
Exercise	−5 mmHg	−4 mmHg
Salt/sodium intake that is moderate or reduced	−5 mmHg on average but greater reductions have been reported in some of the largest clinical trials	−3 mmHg on average but greater reductions have been reported in some of the largest clinical trials
Smoking cessation or any tobacco product (quitting)	No-brainer	No-brainer
Stress reduction	No-brainer	No-brainer
Weight loss of several pounds (2–10% of body weight in overweight individuals)	−3 mmHg	−3 mmHg

Blood Sugar Drugs and Supplements

| Dr. B.S.

"Type II diabetes medications save lives and may help with weight loss."

| Dr. Moyad's No B.S.

"Whatever! Of course type II diabetes medications save lives for the people who qualify for them, but if we were able to really apply the Moyad 23 steps or simple and consistent behavioral changes to many individuals on these medications, it would be wonderful how many millions of people would no longer need these drugs or would just use a lower dosage. Regardless, cardiovascular disease is the number-one cause of death in diabetics, and amputation, blindness, and kidney failure are also real and constant concerns in diabetics, so what more can I say?"

Drugs that control blood sugar for type II diabetes or for those at risk for this disease are critical for the people that need them. While discussing them with your doctor, inquire as to which ones are available in generic form.

Following the 23 steps will help reduce the risk and progression of type II diabetes. For example, eating more healthy fats such as in healthy cooking oils, nuts, seeds, and fish or getting more dietary fiber may actually increase insulin levels or insulin sensitivity and help to maintain normal blood levels of sugar. All these things will also make you heart healthy. *Exercise and belly fat loss are the most powerful lifestyle medications* I have ever seen when individuals want to either go off medication for type II diabetes or just maintain (not increase) or reduce their dosage.

The manufacturers of many dietary supplements have made claims of increasing insulin sensitivity and improving sugar levels or dropping sugar levels, but most of these have a minimal impact and generally only work in individuals with diabetes (not healthy individuals with no blood sugar issues). However, American ginseng has some very minimal evidence and so does chromium (from brewer's yeast sources), cinnamon powder, coccinia indica extract (an herbal product from India also known as coccinia cordifolia), and vanadium dietary supplements. You should be careful about any supplement that causes hypoglycemia or low blood sugar, because dosage is relative, which means some companies have a product that affects your blood sugar at a low dose and some at a higher dose! So, always *start low and go slow with any pill/medication!* However, I do not want you to leave this section without realizing that caffeine sources such as coffee or tea (such as green tea and others) and even the consumption of non-caffeine sources such as moderate amounts of alcohol also have some preliminary evidence that they may reduce the risk of diabetes.

Bone-Loss (Bisphosphonates ...) or Osteoporosis-Prevention Prescription Drugs

This area of medicine is in desperate need of being treated with better and safer risk analysis/assessment/screening, diet, dietary supplements, cholesterol lowering, exercise, weight lifting, and vitamin D blood testing before or even after prescription of the drug.

| Dr. B.S.

"Osteoporosis prevention drugs are very effective at preventing bone fractures!"

| Dr. Moyad's No B.S.

"Whatever! Osteoporosis-prevention drugs are very effective at preventing bone fractures, but they are over-hyped, are over-prescribed, and sit in your body for so long that many people can take a periodic drug holiday from them."

| Dr. B.S. #2

"Osteoporosis is a women's disease."

| Dr. Moyad's No B.S.

"Whatever! Women have a higher risk of having a fracture but men have a higher chance of dying from a fracture, so osteoporosis is a women's and men's disease. We need to quit separating preventive medicine into men's and women's health, because it hurts awareness and education. For example, you make heart disease a men's disease and you spend years playing catch-up in women, who now have a higher risk of dying from heart disease compared to men. You make bone loss a women's disease, and now we wonder why the 90 percent of men that need calcium and vitamin D are not getting it."

Osteoporosis- or bone-fracture prevention pills or injectables known as "bisphosphonates" (such as alendronate, ibandronate, risedronate, ...) usually remain in the body or bone for many years after someone stops taking the drug. So, the drug continues to work long after someone stops taking. Postmenopausal women in the latest clinical trial who took alendronate (Fosamax®) orally for 5 years straight and went off the drug for the next 5 years had no greater risk of having a non-spinal fracture compared to women who took the drug for 10-years straight. Most women also did not lose much bone mineral density after stopping the drug for 5 years. Therefore, many women should talk with their doctor about the possibility of stopping their drug for osteoporosis prevention for some time if they have already taken this drug for 5 or more years. Women at a high risk for a clinical spinal or other fracture should continue taking the drug indefinitely.

I am always disappointed by the osteoporosis drug companies that do not stress more obvious healthy recommendations for women and men who go off or even stay on drug therapy after 5 years or for whatever period of time. These individuals need to get very aggressive about lifestyle changes, such as getting weight-bearing exercise several times a week, not smoking, maintaining normal vitamin D blood levels, getting calcium intakes of up to 1,200 to 1,500 mg per day, and lowering cholesterol.

Jaw Bone Problems with Osteoporosis Drugs?

The use of osteoporosis-prevention drugs known as bisphosphonates and an associated increased risk of osteonecrosis (infection) of the jaw (ONJ) has been gaining a lot of attention lately, and patients should discuss this risk with their doctors and the ways to prevent it from happening.

ONJ has occurred in perhaps thousands of patients, and the numbers are growing with greater awareness. Most of the cases have occurred in patients who need larger amounts of these drugs for longer periods of time. For example, most cases have occurred in multiple myeloma or breast cancer patients, and there has been a recent slight increase in prostate cancer patients. One of the biggest risk factors is having a recent dental procedure or dental problem, but in more rare cases there have been reports in patients without dental issues. Even though occurrences of this condition have been reported with short-term use of these drugs (1 month), the majority of patients have experienced an increased risk with a longer duration of treatment (especially beyond 36 months) and from the IV forms of the drug rather than the pill. Symptoms that have been reported with this rare condition include:

- Mouth or facial pain that resembles a toothache or denture sore
- Chronic sinusitis-like features
- Foul-smelling drainage
- Numbness in the upper or lower jaw area
- Some cases report no symptoms but only one or more white or yellow discolored bony exposure areas in the mouth. The most painful area to touch for the patient has been in the soft tissue area around the exposed bone.

What should be done to prevent ONJ in the first place?

- Before beginning any long-term treatment with a bisphosphonate drug, it has been recommended that patients have a complete dental examination and consultation by a dentist and/or an oral surgeon with experience in this area.
- Any needed dental procedures should be done before going on the drug.
- Patients with dentures should actually use soft liners in some cases.
- During bisphosponate treatment, a regular dental examination schedule should be worked out with the doctor. Any dental procedures or implants in the near future should be planned to consider temporary discontinuation of osteoporosis therapy for a period of time before and after the dental procedure, even though we are not really sure if this will help (be safe rather than sorry). The actual period of time determined by the doctor and patient should be based on the very latest research.

What should be done if ONJ occurs?

The drug should be stopped, and antibiotics can be given. Chlorhexidine mouthwash and irrigation of the area may also help. The long-term prognosis of patients with this condition has not been very good. In the largest studies to date, only approximately 5–20 percent of patients experienced improvement or complete healing.

Quick Review: Any patient about to start or already taking any pill (alendronate or Fosamax, ibandronate or Boniva®, and risedronate or Actonel®), or especially IV bisphosphonate drugs (pamidronate or Aredia®, and zoledronic acid or Reclast® or Zometa®), which is the most common class of osteoporosis-prevention drug, should have a discussion with his or her doctor about this condition. This is such a new and surprising side effect that the best information is up-to-date information, because doctors are literally learning more everyday about it and how to possibly prevent and treat it. It is nice to know that *it is a rare condition.*

Parathyroid Hormone (PTH) is a daily hormone injection that patients can give to themselves with a prescription from the doctor. It is the only FDA-approved drug for severe osteoporosis that actually increases bone formation. PTH should only be given for 1–2 years. After this brief treatment period, patients generally need to start another standard drug for osteoporosis. It has not been found to work better when given at the same time as another standard FDA osteoporosis drug. It is also approved for some men with osteoporosis, especially those with low testosterone levels. Calcium and vitamin D supplements should also be taken daily (which is true of all osteoporosis medications), but the amount should be discussed with the doctor.

Calcium & Vitamin D Supplements

Note: By the time you finish this section, I want you to write in your calcium/vitamin D scores (numbers 1 to 4 below).

    1. Your average daily calcium intake from diet (ideal here to work with a nutritionist) _____.

    2. Divide this average daily intake by 2 (e.g., 750 mg by 2 = 375 mg) _____.

    3. Subtract the number you calculated in line 2 from the recommended total calcium amount for your age group (see the table on p. 137) and that number is_____, which is how much you have to *minimally* get from a calcium supplement.

    4. I had a 25-OH vitamin D blood test in the last year and my vitamin D level was ___ ng/ml or ____ nmol/L.

| Dr. B.S. #1

"Calcium and vitamin D do not prevent bone fractures."

| Dr. Moyad's No B.S.

"Whatever! Calcium, vitamin D, weight lifting, and cholesterol lowering do reduce bone fractures as long as you can take your dietary supplement pills (about 80 percent of the time) and exercise regularly. This advice needs to be followed even when taking prescription bone health drugs."

| Dr. B.S. #2

"Expensive calcium supplements work better than cheaper calcium supplements, and vitamin D supplements are not needed if you drink milk or get sun exposure on a regular basis."

| Dr. Moyad's No B.S.

"Whatever! Cheap calcium carbonate and other supplements work as well as the most expensive ones. The dosage and type of calcium supplement you should take should be decided after meeting with a nutritionist to discover how much calcium you initially get from dietary sources, and after discussing your health history with your doctor. Also, the recommended daily allowance for vitamin D should be increased immediately to at least 800 to 1,000 IU per day, and annual vitamin D blood testing (25-OH vitamin D) should be covered by all insurance plans now, or you should try and pay for it out of pocket."

First and foremost, it is critical to determine your calcium and vitamin D requirements. Below is a list of standard government requirements. How are you doing? The recommended daily allowance for calcium is excellent and needs to be applied to men and women. However, the recommended daily allowance for vitamin D is inadequate and should be increased immediately. Everyone should also include yearly or every-other-year blood testing for vitamin D in fall or winter time, when vitamin D production in your body is at its lowest.

Let's review the approximate requirements for total calcium (mg) and vitamin D (in IU or mcg; note every 200 IU of vitamin D equals 5 mcg) daily intake including diet and supplements for women and men. Keep in mind that regardless of the adult age, the average intake of calcium is about 600 mg to 800 mg per day at best. My recommendations for increases in vitamin D are included.

Calcium and Vitamin D Requirements

Age	Calcium (mg)	Vitamin D (IU)
0–6 months	200	200
7–12 months	250	200 or 5 mcg (Moyad 400 or 10 mcg)
1–3 years	500	200 or 5 mcg (Moyad 400 or 10 mcg)
4–8 years	800	200 or 5 mcg (Moyad 400 or 10 mcg)
9–18 years	1,200	200 (Moyad 800–1,000 or 20–25 mcg)
19–50 years	1,000	200 (Moyad 800–1,000 or 20–25 mcg)
50–70 years	1,200	400 (Moyad 800–1,000 or 20–25 mcg)
Over 70 years	1,200	600 (Moyad 800–1,000 or 20 –25 mcg)
Pregnancy	1,200	400 (Moyad 800–1000 or 20–25 mcg)
Lactation	1,200	400 (Moyad 800–1000 or 20–25 mcg)

Sources: Surgeon General's Report on Bone Health and Osteoporosis and National Academy of Sciences.

Here is how to think about it: when you hit the age of ten, you should generally get about or at least 1,000 mg of calcium a day *total* (from diet and supplements) and close to 1,000 IU of vitamin D (from diet and supplements after being blood tested in the fall or winter) *for the rest of your life regardless of whether you are a woman or man.*

Now it is time to take a look at the foods and beverages listed below in order to understand how much of your daily calcium intake may be coming from healthy foods and beverages.

Approximate Calcium Content of Some Low-Saturated-Fat Foods

Dietary Item	Calcium Amount (mg per 3.5 ounce or 100 gram serving)
Kelp	1,100
Collards	360
Orange juice (fortified)	350
Sardines	325
Oatmeal (instant)	325
Yogurt	300
Milk	300
Figs (dried)	270
Cheese	270
Kale	250
Spinach	244
Almonds	235
Brewer's yeast	210
Parsley	205
Brazil nuts	185
Soybeans	175
Watercress	150
Tofu	130
Sunflower seeds	120
Broccoli	105
Olives (ripe)	105
Beans (other)	50–100
Nuts (other)	50–100
Cottage cheese	95
Brussels sprouts	55
Orange	55

Raisins	50
Brown rice	50
Carrots	35

Now, the bad news—most of the calcium that you get from foods or beverages is not absorbed well by the human body. Therefore, when determining the range of calcium intake needed, keep in mind that only about 33–50 percent of the total calcium listed in the items above and from other food/beverage sources is actually absorbed. This is why many doctors tell their patients to get some of their daily calcium requirements from dietary supplements.

So, after you are able to determine your absorbed dietary calcium intake, you should make up for the difference with dietary supplements. For example, my daily calcium intake is about 800 to 900 mg per day (on a good day), so I take one calcium carbonate supplement per day. Calcium supplements are not only generally safe but are effective at reducing the risk of fractures. *But, if they are not taken regularly (about 24–25 days of every month), they simply do not work in many cases.*

Two recent randomized controlled studies of calcium supplements need to be reviewed, because the public has been waiting 5–10 years for the results. The first study was the Women's Health Initiative (WHI), and the second was from the University of Western Australia (UWA). The overall findings of the two studies are summarized in the table below.

Summary of the UWA and WHI Calcium Supplement Clinical Trials

	University of Western Australia (UWA) Study	Women's Health Initiative (WHI) Study
Average age	75	62
Number of participants	1,460	36,000
Average length of the study	5 years	7 years
Dosage of calcium used in the study	1,200 mg/day of calcium carbonate	1,000 mg/day of calcium carbonate + 400 IU/day of vitamin D3

	University of Western Australia (UWA) Study	Women's Health Initiative (WHI) Study
Overall benefit in terms of reducing fractures	None	None
Percentage of women who took their calcium pills regularly (80% or more of their tablets)	57%	59%
The fracture risk reduction observed in the regular pill takers	34% reduction in total fractures, and 56% reduction in upper limb fractures	29% reduction in hip fractures
Side effects	Constipation (13.4% compared to 9.1% in the placebo group; only side effect difference compared to placebo out of over 92,000 claims of side effects in the trial.)	Kidney stones (17% increased risk; dietary intake before the trial does not impact the risk of stones, and lower intakes of calcium may have actually increased the risk of a kidney stone)
Other important findings	900 to 950 mg/day of calcium from dietary sources was also consumed in addition to supplementation	Women that were physically active also seemed to reduce their risk of fractures.

Note: The conclusion of the UWA study was well stated: "However, these data support the continued use of calcium supplements by women who are able to remain compliant with their use. In these individuals, especially if they are under the care of a clinician, calcium supplementation is a safe and effective therapy for reducing the risk of osteoporotic fracture." In other words, for women and even men compliance or regularly taking required supplements or medication is the key to reducing the risk of certain conditions that can actually be life-threatening. This was remarkably similar to the conclusion of the U.S. WHI clinical trial. In other words, compliance is the key to calcium supplements and an improvement in bone health.

Choosing a Calcium Supplement

I like the calcium supplements, but before a commercial gets to you, please make sure that you learn about the positives and negatives of each product. In general, the higher percentage of elemental calcium by weight, the more beneficial the product.

Type of Calcium Supplement*	Elemental Calcium by Weight	Moyad No B.S. Comments
Calcium carbonate	40% (less pills to take to achieve your goal)	My first choice: most tested; requires fewest pills/day; can be used as an acid reflux drug. Least expensive Should be taken with food because you need some stomach acid to absorb these supplements, in general.
Calcium citrate or Calcium citrate malate	21%	My third choice: better absorbed, especially in a low-acid stomach environment so it can be taken with or without food. More expensive & more pills needed daily, so long-term compliance is an issue.
Calcium phosphate	38% or 31%	My second choice: fewer pills to take, in general. Tricalcium or dicalcium phosphate Can be taken with or without food. Simplicity and price getting closer to calcium carbonate. Needs many more clinical trials before they will be recommended on a regular basis.

*Ideally, calcium dietary supplements should be taken in divided doses throughout the day, because the human body generally absorbs approximately 500 mg of elemental calcium at a time. If you happen to take more than this at once, do not sweat it because you will still absorb some of both supplements. Check for the amount of "elemental calcium" in each tablet, because this is the form of calcium that is absorbed and actually counted for the required daily calcium intake for women and men. Some of the above supplements may also contain vitamin D, which increases capsule/tablet size just a little. You may want to get vitamin D from a separate supplement or source in order to reduce the size of the pill you are taking. You do not need to have vitamin D in your calcium supplement for better absorption (B.S. myth of major proportions). Vitamin D is a fat-soluble vitamin that takes months to deplete and does *not* have to be in your calcium supplement.

Vitamin D

Let's talk about the number-one deficiency of any vitamin or mineral in the United States, regardless of age, gender, race, color, creed— Vitamin D.

The Primary Factors That Can Determine Vitamin D Levels

Factor	Comment
Aging	Older individuals make less vitamin D for many reasons: 7-dehydrocholesterol in the skin is lower, so it is more difficult to make vitamin D3 (e.g., individuals above the age of 65 have a fourfold reduction in the capacity of the skin to produce vitamin D3); liver & kidney function is not as efficient; & the stomach's ability to absorb vitamin D from food or supplements is reduced.
Belly fat	Obese individuals tend to have lower vitamin D concentrations because this vitamin gets absorbed by fat tissue and is not easily released in the blood stream (more fat = less available vitamin D).
Cholesterol-lowering medications (statins)	Preliminary research suggests that lowering cholesterol may increase vitamin D levels
Dietary vitamin D intake (natural or non-fortified sources)	The more vitamin D one gets from dietary sources, the higher the blood level. Fish are the best dietary source, followed by much lower amounts in mushrooms and egg yolks.

Dietary vitamin D intake (fortified vitamin D sources)	In the U.S. and Canada, milk, soy milk, bread products, cereals, protein bars, and other foods & beverages are fortified with vitamin D. In Europe, margarine is one of the more common fortified sources of vitamin D. Independent surveys have found that many of these products do not contain the amount of vitamin D on the label (usually less).
Intake frequency of vitamin D	Recent research has demonstrated that taking a daily pill has a better chance of keeping a normal blood level of vitamin D compared to a once–a–week or once-a-month formulation.
Skin pigmentation	Darker-skinned individuals have more melanin (increased skin pigmentation) that blocks the impact of UV-B radiation and reduces the production of vitamin D. African-American individuals have a higher risk of vitamin D deficiency.
Sunlight exposure	The more your occupation or activities involve being outdoors, especially in the spring and summer, the greater the chance that you will have higher vitamin D levels.
Sunscreen/Sun-protective clothing	The higher the SPF of your sunscreen, the more it blocks the ability of UV-B light from the sun and reduces vitamin D production. This is also the case with sun-protective clothing
Supplemental vitamin D	Multivitamins generally contain 400 IU (10 mcg)/capsule. Many of these pills and liquids contain vitamin D2 and not the Moyad-preferred vitamin D3 form.
Ultraviolet-B (UV-B) light radiation (wavelength = 290–315 nm) exposure based on where you live	UV-B radiation from the sun is the primary source of vitamin D for most people. Thus, geographic location/how much sunlight affects how much vitamin D you produce (more sun or closer to the equator = more vitamin D). Above and below latitudes of approx. 40 degrees north and south, vitamin D production in skin hardly occurs in the winter (Boston, MA is 42 degrees north & Edmonton, Canada is 53 degrees)

The only foods that naturally contain vitamin D are seafood/fish (good source, and I find it interesting such a heart-healthy food contains the highest natural source of vitamin D), mushrooms (small source), and egg yolks (small source).

Food	Serving Size	Vitamin D (IU)
Oysters	3 oz.	545
Salmon (wild)	3 oz.	1,000
Cod-liver oil	1 teaspoon	450
Catfish	3 oz.	425
Bluefish	3 oz.	415
Mackerel	3 oz.	395
Trout (farmed)	3 oz.	375
Salmon (farmed)	3 oz.	275
Sardines (canned in oil)	3 oz.	230
Halibut	3 oz.	170
Tuna (bluefin)	3 oz.	170
Tuna (canned in water)	3 oz.	135
Shrimp	3 oz.	120
Milk*	1 cup	100
Cod	3 oz.	80
Mushrooms (shitake)	2 oz.	55
Mushrooms (chanterelle)	2 oz.	50
Sole/flounder	3 oz.	50
Bass (freshwater)	3 oz.	35
Swordfish	3 oz.	35
Clams	3 oz.	30
Egg (whole)	1	25

*Whole, low-fat, or non-fat/skim milk is supposed to be fortified with 100 IU of vitamin D per cup, but past studies have not yet definitely proven the reliability of the fortification process. Studies have suggested that many dairy products are under-fortified with vitamin D, despite claims on the labels.

In some countries vitamin D is listed in micrograms, so here is the relationship.

- 2.5 mcg (micrograms) = 100 IU
- 5 mcg = 200 IU
- 10 mcg = 400 IU
- 15 mcg = 600 IU
- 20 mcg = 800 IU

What is the best type of vitamin D to take?

There are basically two types of vitamin D supplements available for over-the-counter purchase—Vitamin D2 and Vitamin D3, but vitamin D3 (not vitamin D2) is the type that most experts believe should be taken. I am just happy that anyone gets vitamin D from the diet and supplements, so even if it is vitamin D2 this is good, but eventually a person should switch to D3.

Let's review the case for vitamin D3.

- Sunshine hits the human body, and we make vitamin D3. It is the most natural form. Humans do not make vitamin D2.
- Wild fish have mostly vitamin D3 and not vitamin D2, but farmed fish seem to have higher levels of vitamin D2.
- Vitamin D3 is as cheap as vitamin D2.
- Vitamin D3 may be less toxic than D2, because higher concentrations of D2 circulate in the blood when taken (compared to vitamin D3). Vitamin D2 does not bind as well to the receptors in the human tissues compared to vitamin D3.
- Vitamin D3 is the more potent form of vitamin D. This is a potential benefit because obesity tends to lower blood levels of vitamin D, so a more potent form is needed.
- Vitamin D3 is more stable on the shelf than D2 and is more likely to remain active for a longer period of time when exposed to different conditions (temperature, humidity, and storage). In numerous cases, this is why the amount of vitamin D2 in certain food products has been different from that advertised on the label.
- Vitamin D3 has been the most studied type of vitamin D in clinical trials. There have only been a few clinical trials of vitamin D2 to prevent bone fractures in adults.
- Vitamin D3 is more effective at raising and *maintaining* the results of the vitamin D blood test.

Vitamin D2 is a plant- or fungus/yeast–derived product, and it was first produced in the early 1920s by exposing foods to ultraviolet light. This process was patented and licensed to pharmaceutical companies. To this day, many prescription forms of vitamin D are actually vitamin D2 and not vitamin D3. Multivitamins have either vitamin D2 or D3, but many companies are now making the switch to D3. Numerous past clinical studies dating back almost 50 to 100 years continue to suggest that vitamin D3 may be about two to ten times as potent as vitamin D2.

When buying vitamin D, please purchase vitamin D3 (also known as "cholecalciferol" on the label) instead of vitamin D2 (also known as "ergocalciferol" on the label), because vitamin D3 is not expensive and is the most clinically studied, the least toxic, and the most natural form of vitamin D for humans. However, I do not want to B.S. you into thinking that vitamin D2 is not effective, because it is, and so is the injectable form of vitamin D that is given by some doctors for patients who have a tough time taking pills.

How much vitamin D do you really need?

About 800 to 1,000 IU per day or what you and your doctor decide after you get a blood test during the fall through wintertime (when blood levels of vitamin D are at their lowest). Most people should have a vitamin D blood level of 35–40 ng/ml (90–100 nmol/L).

In the 1970s the test for vitamin D known as "25-OH vitamin D" was invented. This test would eventually show that it reflects the amount of vitamin D in the body that was coming from all sources (diet, dietary supplements, and the sun), which is why the test is so wonderful. In addition, researchers found that a low concentration of 25-OH vitamin D causes secondary hyperparathyroidism (high levels of parathyroid hormone or PTH), which means a person loses more calcium from the bones when PTH is abnormally high and has an even greater risk for bone loss.

Now you know why in the past few decades, the best blood level of vitamin D (25-OH vitamin D) was based on the amount needed to keep the hormone known as parathyroid hormone (PTH) from getting abnormally high. Since PTH at high levels can cause calcium loss from the bone, it would make sense that vitamin D could maintain or improve bone health at these levels. However, PTH can change due to kidney function, exercise level, the time of day, or even the diet. So, there has been no consensus on the optimal level of vitamin

D intake to reduce PTH, and this is why many laboratories report that the normal range of vitamin D varies as much as 20 to 40 ng/ml in some cases to 20 to 100 nmol in other cases. So, what is the best blood level of vitamin D?

Several prominent experts put together a review of a large number of past studies in order to arrive at an answer to this question. And I could not agree more with the findings. They evaluated a variety of health changes, not just bone health. They also wanted to know what vitamin D level could maintain muscle strength, prevent falls, improve dental health, and prevent cancer (especially colorectal cancer). Other claims for vitamin D that are not as strong include preventing multiple sclerosis, insulin problems (diabetes), other cancers, arthritis, hypertension, and tuberculosis. They also looked at a variety of other things apart from keeping PTH normal, and looked at studies in a variety of ethnic groups. These experts ended up coming back to the same consistent answer—most studies in a variety of health areas point toward a blood level of vitamin D that is between 90 to 100 nmol/L or 35 to 40 ng/ml for preventive health. *This means most people would need to take about 800 to 1,000 IU (or more) to achieve a normal blood level of vitamin D.*

Keep in mind that, in general, 100 IU (2.5 mcg) of vitamin D/day can raise your blood test about 1 ng/ml after 2 to 3 months. So, let's review this important question for you and your doctor, namely how much vitamin D do I need per day in order to get my vitamin D blood test to a normal level in two to three months?

- 100 IU (2.5 mcg) per day increases vitamin D blood levels 1 ng/ml (2.5 nmol/L)
- 200 IU (5 mcg) per day increases vitamin D blood levels 2 ng/ml (5 nmol/L)
- 400 IU (10 mcg) per day increases vitamin D blood levels 4 ng/ml (10 nmol/L)
- 500 IU (12.5 mcg) per day increases vitamin D blood levels 5 ng/ml (12.5 nmol/L)
- 800 IU (20 mcg) per day increases vitamin D blood levels 8 ng/ml (20 nmol/L)
- 1000 IU (25 mcg) per day increases vitamin D blood levels 10 ng/ml (25 nmol/L)
- 2000 IU (50 mcg) per day increases vitamin D blood levels 20 ng/ml (50 nmol/L)

As an example, if your vitamin D blood test was 30 ng/ml (75 nmol/L) and you wanted to get to 40 ng/ml (100 nmol/L), you would need to take 1,000 IU (25 mcg) of vitamin D/day over several months in order to get to a normal blood level or 40 ng/ml (100 nmol/L).

What about side effects?

Some studies have given healthy individuals 100,000 IU vitamin D3 tablets every 4 months compared to a placebo, and it was an interesting study because it involved mostly doctors as the participants. This turned out to be a safe level.

Toxicity has not been established. A 21-year old man or woman exposed to summer UV-B light generates 10,000 IU (the equivalent of 250 mcg or 25 multivitamin pills of vitamin D or 100 glasses of milk) of vitamin D in 15–20 minutes, but longer exposure does not produce more. So, humans were basically built to produce and carry higher levels of vitamin D when exposed to the sun.

It is also important to mention that the experiences of this expert vitamin D group suggest that higher vitamin D levels are safe. Previous research suggests that the first sign of real side effects or toxicity of vitamin D occurs at a blood level of greater than 88 ng/ml (220 nmol/L), where abnormally high blood levels of calcium result from too much absorption of calcium from food, and that can lead to problems. Regardless, stick with 40ng/ml (100 nmol/L) as your target.

Let's finish this discussion by looking at the forest beyond the tree and why I think calcium and vitamin D pills need to be discussed with every individual.

A Partial List of the Overall (Mostly Non-Osteoporosis) Potential Health Benefits of Consuming Recommended Amounts of Dietary or Supplemental Calcium and/or Vitamin D

Health Condition	Calcium	Vitamin D
Acid reflux	Calcium carbonate is a natural antacid.	No impact
Arthritis/muscle pain	May reduce the impact	May reduce the impact
Bone loss & Muscle strength/coordination	We know it reduces the risk of bone loss & fractures.	We know it reduces the risk of bone loss & fractures & improves muscle strength.

Cardiovascular disease (CVD)	May reduce	May reduce
Cholesterol, especially HDL (good cholesterol)	May increase HDL	Unknown
Cancer & colon polyps	May reduce the risk of recurrent colon polyps & may lower the risk of colon & other cancers.	Evidence suggests a lower risk of colon and other cancers.
Dental hygiene	May reduce the risk of tooth loss	May reduce the risk of tooth loss
Diabetes (type I)	Unknown	May reduce the risk of type I diabetes in children
Hypertension (high blood pressure)	May lower blood pressure in hypertensive individuals.	May reduce the risk of high blood pressure.
Kidney stones (calcium oxalate)	May prevent calcium oxalate stones.	Unknown
Lung function & Lung disease	Unknown	May improve lung function in asthmatics & may reduce the risk of lung disease.
Multiple sclerosis	Unknown	May reduce the risk of multiple sclerosis & other autoimmune diseases.
Obesity	May stimulate lipolysis (fat breakdown) in obese patients and reduce weight, but this is controversial.	Unknown, but may slightly reduce weight; excessive intake may encourage weight gain.
Pregnancy	May improve the bone health of the baby when taken by the mother.	May improve the bone health of the baby when taken by the mother & should be studied in the area of autism prevention

Health Condition	Calcium	Vitamin D
Premenstrual syndrome (PMS) symptoms	May reduce symptoms of PMS	Unknown
Prostate health	May decrease the PSA blood test (not sure if this is real or an artificial decrease)	May decrease the PSA blood test (not sure if this is real or an artificial decrease)

I am *not* suggesting that calcium and vitamin D are the solutions to most health problems. I get nervous about just relying on a pill. It is possible that as a society relies more on higher doses of some components while ignoring the overall health benefits of other components of diet and lifestyle, there is an overall deleterious impact. We need to remember that numerous healthy changes are superior to only a few changes in excess. It is interesting that in countries that have higher rates of bone fractures, there also exist higher rates of cardiovascular disease and possibly other chronic conditions. Again, disease prevention in many cases seems to be intimately related across multiple conditions, and not mutually exclusive. The specific and generally agreed-upon anti-osteoporosis lifestyle changes and supplements seem to be similar, for the most part, to the anti–heart disease, anti–breast cancer, anti–colon cancer, anti–prostate cancer, anti–kidney stone, etc. recommendations, and this is the important point that must be emphasized.

Whether or not you should take calcium and vitamin D supplements is dependent on whether or not you qualify for these pills. To see if you qualify for calcium supplements, you should ideally determine how much calcium you get from dietary sources working with a nutritionist, and to see how much vitamin D you need you should work with the blood test and your doctor.

Cholesterol-Lowering Drugs and Supplements

| Dr. B.S. #1

"Statin drugs are dangerous and should be avoided because they cause muscle and liver problems."

| Dr. Moyad's No B.S.

"Whatever! If people really understood the research on statin drugs, they would not hesitate to at least try them, and they would generally feel as comfortable taking them as any vitamin or over-the-counter product! Statins are simply one of the greatest overall preventive pills of my lifetime, and everyone should have a discussion with their doctor about them and to see if they *qualify* for one!"

| Dr. B.S. #2

"Hey, I take _____ statin drug because it is the best and I am a doctor!"

| Dr. Moyad's No B.S.

"Research has clearly demonstrated that the cost and the type of statin drug have nothing to do with the overall clinical benefits. Whatever statin pill allows you to reach your targeted cholesterol goal with your doctor, and whatever pill you see as the easiest to take over years and years that is reasonably priced or covered by your insurance plan is the best one to take for you!"

| Dr. B.S. #3

"Wait for more results on Vytorin® (a combination of a statin with a cholesterol absorption blocking pill) before we decide to replace it with another drug, Mr. or Ms. or Mrs. ..."

| Dr. Moyad's No B.S.

"Actually you need to think about going off Vytorin or Zetia® right now, at least until the drugs prove themselves to be as safe and as good as the standard statin medications. Personally, I would not take either medication right now until we get more positive research that makes clinical sense about these medications."

The amazing thing about cholesterol-lowering drugs is that they not only seem to reduce the risk of cardiovascular disease, but also have recently been associated with a lower risk of numerous cancers and possibly dying from some types of cancer. They may even improve your prognosis during and after treatment for some cancers. If I am wrong about this thought, well at least these medications still reduce the number-one cause of death in women and men (cardiovascular disease).

If you cannot get your cholesterol down to the normal levels, do not be shy about asking your doctor about going on a statin drug or another cholesterol-lowering drug or another heart-healthy drug.

Dr. Moyad, what about muscle and joint aches?

There is no relationship between the dosage of a cholesterol-lowering drug (statin) and muscle and joint aches. In other words, it can occur at any dosage and at any time, but overall this is not a common occurrence. A common and popular way to reduce muscle and joint problems with a statin is to take 50–100 mg a day of coenzyme Q10 supplements. Some people experience a reduction in muscle and joint problems with these supplements. However, do not take this supplement with your statin without consulting with your doctor.

Dr. Moyad, what about liver problems when taking statins?

There is a direct relationship between liver problems and the dosage of the statin drug. The higher dosages of the statin, the greater the risk of liver problems, but again, this is a rare event, and doctors have an easy blood test to detect any problems. Therefore, the biggest reason in my opinion people run into problems with statins is that they do not maintain their medical appointments.

Statins have been so safe that in certain parts of the world, some low-dose statins are actually sold over the counter. In my opinion, low-dose statins are actually safer than baby aspirin for some individuals.

All statins work better at night except Crestor® and Lipitor®, which can be taken at any time. These two drugs remain in the blood for the longest period of time in this drug class. In reality, it is still okay in my opinion to take a statin drug at any time because taking something daily for most of your life is not easy.

Also, Crestor and Lipitor have been taken every other day or once every 3–4 days by some patients, and they have achieved the same numerical results in my opinion. This is an option for a small number of patients who have trouble taking these drugs. However, all statin drugs have the option of being taken every other day or once every few days if there is a problem with taking them daily.

When an LDL ("bad cholesterol")–lowering drug or statin is used, the dosage needed to reduce LDL between 30 and 40 percent is a good way to compare effective dosages.

Statin Drug	Dose (mg/day)	LDL Reduction (%)
Atorvastatin (Lipitor)	10	39
Fluvastatin (Lescol®)	40-80	25–35
Lovastatin (Mevacor®) (less expensive)	40	31
Pravastatin (Pravachol®) (less expensive and researched with numerous clinical studies)	40	34
Rosuvastatin (Crestor)	5–10	39–45
Simvastatin (Zocor®) (less expensive)	20–40	35–41

Now, let's review the statin drugs one more time, but in a more practical, personal, realistic, and evidence-based way.

- Atorvastatin (Lipitor) is a great drug with very effective marketing, and one of the most potent statin drugs that I trust right now. A drawback is that it has not been well studied in the area of preventive medicine (people who are completely healthy) or in people who have never had cardiovascular disease.
- Fluvastatin (Lescol) is a very effective drug, but has received very little research, so it is my least favorite.
- Lovastatin (Mevacor) has lost its patent and is dirt cheap, so it is a wonderful option for those on a tight budget.
- Pravachol (Pravastatin) is one of my favorites because of cost (also has lost its patent), and it has been studied in some of the biggest preventive trials where people did not have heart disease and were completely healthy when taking it. The study reported few side effects and many benefits. Also, it is the only statin that is not heavily metabolized by the liver, so people seem to have fewer side effect issues with this drug.
- Rosuvastatin (Crestor) is the most powerful statin drug, which means it has the biggest impact on your cholesterol numbers when comparing statin doses head to head. It is also the statin drug that increases your HDL or "good cholesterol" the most!

However, it is not cheap and has not received enough clinical trials, but its future looks promising in terms of reducing hs-CRP and preventing heart disease.

- Simvastatin (Zocor) by itself is a wonderful statin drug because it has lost its patent and is cheap, and it has been very well studied. Recently, it has even been combined with Zetia (another pill) to create Vytorin, which is another cholesterol-lowering agent. However, the only problem with Vytorin is the Zetia part of the pill, because this has not been well studied. Vytorin is not a good drug in my opinion and should not be taken until Vytorin or Zetia has proven itself to be worthy of taking ... it is that simple.
- Red-yeast rice extract (from China generally, also known as "Monascus Purpureus") dietary supplements have been available on the U.S. market for several years. Currently they have been involved in litigation because some companies argue that this natural supplement has a similar structure to cholesterol-lowering drugs (statins). They do some have similarities to the statin drugs (especially lovastatin), which means they are probably effective. The problem is that you and your doctor have to guess how effective they are because the companies are not allowed to standardize the amount of the active statin-like ingredient in the dietary supplement. Some of the research shows that anywhere from 600 to 2,400 mg of the stuff daily works. If you want to try it, pick up a red-yeast rice extract brand from a reputable company and start working with your doctor because this supplement should work. The downside is that you have to pay completely out of pocket for it compared to the other statins, which may be covered by your insurance. Another downside is that it looks and acts like a statin, but it has never proven itself to be as good as a statin.

The overall impact of a variety of statins on the most important clinical events, such as reducing the risk of death, heart attacks, and strokes, is identical. In other words, one drug is no better than the other drug as long as the right cholesterol number is achieved. Regardless of what the fancy commercials tell you, these drugs all work equally well as long as the appropriate dosage is used.

There are many other ways to reduce cholesterol with a pill, including fibrate drugs (if triglycerides are a problem), e.g., fenofibrate (or Tricor®). Niacin is also an option and is probably the best drug ever invented to safely increase HDL or "good cholesterol" levels. Niacin (nicotinic acid) comes in several forms:

- Immediate-release crystalline niacin or the over-the counter-version work as well, with a higher rate of hot flashes as a side effect, and a lower risk of liver problems.
- Extended-release niacin (Niaspan®), which is a prescription drug, also works well and may be covered by insurance. It has a moderate risk of hot flashes and liver problems.
- Lovastatin/niacin-extended-release (Advicor®) is a prescription combination of Niaspan and the first statin or cholesterol-lowering drug ever sold, Lovastatin.
- Sustained-release (or time-released) niacin, which can be purchased over the counter, has the highest risk of liver problems, and most people should never take this form.
- There is a new simvastatin (Zocor)/niacin combination drug (should be known as SIMCOR®) that should be available. You can ask your doctor about this one if you are interested.
- No-flush niacin does not cause a flush but it is not as effective.

The secret to niacin and reducing its side effects is to take the pills with a full meal, or take an aspirin (if you qualify) about 15–30 minutes before you take the niacin to reduce the hot flash side effects. Another secret is to start with a lower dosage daily for at least one month and then increase your dose if needed, because the human body develops tolerance or naturally begins to adjust to niacin over time, and the hot flash side effects begin to become less severe over time in many people.

Dr. Moyad, the statin drugs are not natural, so I am nervous about taking them. What do you think?

Never be fooled by the marketing of the natural versus synthetic debate. Arsenic and cyanide are natural products, but you do not see me taking them. The first three statins invented (Mevacor, Pravachol, and Zocor) came from a fungus! Also, red-yeast rice extract is the natural source of a statin, but it is more diluted, so it does not work as well as a statin.

Who wins? Aspirin versus a statin for overall health?

In my opinion, if cost was not an issue this discussion would not be an issue. When comparing a statin to aspirin to prevent a first cardiovascular event in men or women, aspirin is not necessarily better; it is just cheaper.

Whether or not to take aspirin after a first heart attack or even to take a statin after such an event is not an issue. This is standard medicine. However, what is more confusing is whether or not to take an aspirin and/or statin to reduce the risk of a first cardiac event or heart attack. It is interesting that there are no national guidelines for the recommendation of aspirin versus a statin or for when the two should be combined to prevent a first cardiovascular disease (CVD) event (also known as primary prevention). A recent study published by several experts attempted to answer this question. After reviewing all of the studies they concluded that aspirin is cheaper and more effective for preventing CVD events in middle-aged (a 45-year-old who does not smoke) men whose 10-year risk for heart disease is 7.5 percent or higher, and adding a statin to aspirin becomes more cost effective when an individual's 10-year risk is higher than 10 percent. In other words, adding a statin becomes more cost-effective as risk increases. I think this advice should be true for women.

A closer look at this analysis revealed some interesting findings. When the authors of this study compared the data from all of the primary prevention trials in men, a summary of what they found is listed in the table.

Statin Versus Aspirin for the Prevention of Cardiovascular Disease (CVD), and Other Benefits and Risks of Using Either Drug Alone

Specific Event Being Studied in a Primary Prevention (Healthy Population) Setting	Statin	Aspirin
Heart attack (also known as myocardial infarction)	Reduced risk by 30%	Reduced risk by 30%
Stroke	Reduced risk by 15%	No impact (actually may increase the risk of hemorrhagic stroke but lowers the risk of an ischemic stroke in older and higher risk people)

Angina (chest pain)	Reduced risk by 72%	No impact
Death from coronary heart disease	Reduced risk by 29%	Reduced risk by 13%
Myopathy or muscle problems	Occurs in 1 out of 1,000 users of statins annually	No risk of myopathy
Death because of myopathy	Occurs in 1 out of 100,000 users of statins annually	No risk of death from myopathy
Gastrointestinal bleeding that usually requires a transfusion (includes peptic ulcers)	No risk of bleeding	Occurs in 7 out of 10,000 users of aspirin annually
Death from gastrointestinal bleeding	No risk of death	Occurs in 1 out of 100,000 users of aspirin annually
Hemorrhagic or bleeding stroke	No risk of hemorrhagic stroke	20 hemorrhagic strokes per 100,000 users of aspirin annually
Miscellaneous health benefits/side effects	Has been associated with a lower risk of many cancers, many types of cardiovascular disease, eye disease, neurologic diseases, and dying young from any cause. Very low cholesterol numbers need more research into whether or not they reduce short-term memory.*	May reduce the risk of colon polyps, but this is now controversial. Is not associated with memory problems.
Cost	Moderate, but getting cheaper by the day!	Cheap

*The controversy on whether or not a statin or dosage that reduces your cholesterol by a gigantic amount (for example to an LDL far below 70 points in the American system) may actually also reduce your short-term memory is receiving research right now. I am sure that having a cholesterol level that is far below your targeted goal cannot be healthy for some individuals, because everything works in moderation and the brain needs a certain amount of cholesterol and fat in the diet to function.

Looking at the above table creates a different picture from what the authors offer, in my opinion. Statins seem to reduce the risk of heart attacks, stroke, angina, and deaths from heart disease as well as if not better than aspirin. When it comes to side effects, there is a higher risk of muscle problems and death from muscle problems in statin users, but in aspirin users there is a higher risk of bleeding and dying from internal bleeding! Some doctors favor aspirin use first although the statin seems to work better, but because of cost many experts favor aspirin use first and then add a statin as risk of CVD increases. This is surprising, because many people can afford statins today, and in 2006 there were three different statins that lost their patents (Mevacor, Pravachol, and Zocor), which means the prices of these drugs as a whole should continue to drop! Also, it should be kept in mind that myopathy or muscle problems from a statin are not only reversible in most cases when you quit the drug, but also detectable by a blood test that monitors the risk of muscle problems (the CPK blood test). Bleeding from aspirin internally has no test that helps clinicians predict with good accuracy whether or not this will happen.

Please remember: Heart Healthy = All Healthy
and Heart Unhealthy = All Unhealthy!

Fish Oil (Omega-3) Supplements

| Dr. B.S.

"High-priced fish oil supplements, including the prescription form, have the best quality control, so they are clearly worth the price!"

| Dr. Moyad's No B.S.

"Whatever! Fish oil dietary supplements used in clinical trials and sold throughout the world mostly come from low-priced anchovies and sardines. Their inherent small size (meaning little to no mercury and other contaminants) and high omega-3 content do not make quality control an issue in most cases. Consequently, higher-priced fish oil pills are not any better than some of the medium- or low-priced fish oil pills in terms of safety and clinical effects. Everyone should talk to a doctor about whether or not they qualify for them. Fish oil pills were one of the only over-the-counter pills to first establish themselves as heart healthy, mentally healthy, and safe in pregnancy in moderation before they were touted and tested in other areas. However, if people tell you there are absolutely no side effects of fish oil pills when taking large doses, please tell them they are full of B.S."

You know an over-the-counter pill makes money and is healthy if there is a prescription version also available. For example, niacin is a wonderful supplement, but it also comes in a high-dose prescription form! And now there is the omega-3 prescription known as Lovaza®. In general, one of the prescription pills is equal to 2–3 over-the-counter pills in terms of omega-3 amount. In my opinion, the only advantage to the expensive prescription omega-3 pill is simply the number of pills you have to take compared to the over-the-counter pill.

The most common fish oil pills or capsules in the United States today provide 180 mg of EPA and 120 mg of DHA per capsule, which means 300 mg of the active ingredient (in a 1 gram or 1,000 mg fish oil capsule). I also like fish oil or omega-3 pills for heart disease prevention that have almost equivalent amounts of EPA and DHA, whereas in pregnancy having equal amounts or more of DHA than EPA is okay. The point is that I do not like pills with only one type of omega-3 fatty acid in them (like DHA), because this does not follow the best research. Remember, there are 3 omega-3 compounds that have clinical evidence and they are ALA, EPA, and DHA.

Keep in mind that even fish oils come with a catch. They may thin your blood too much and increase your risk of internal bleeding. Please discuss with your doctor whether or not you qualify for a fish oil supplement. Obviously, individuals already on another blood thinning medication have to be careful when combining it with fish oil pills.

Other areas of medicine are getting a lot of attention with fish oil or omega-3.

Partial Summary of the Potential Diverse Medical Benefits of Omega-3 Fatty Acids from Laboratory, Epidemiologic, and Clinical Studies

Medical Specialty (Which omega-3—ALA, EPA, or DHA—has the most supporting evidence?)	Potential Reduction in Risk or Impact/Comment
Cardiology (ALA, EPA & DHA) Note: If you have had a medical procedure where they gave you a pacemaker or have given you an ICD (implantable cardioverter-defibrillator), please do not take omega-3 pills until you have asked your doctor about the latest research of whether these pills help, hurt, or have no impact.	ALA, EPA & DHA all have some evidence to suggest they lower the risk of dying early from heart disease and lower the risk of sudden cardiac death, irregular heart beats or rhythms & ischemic strokes, and these compounds may also lower heart rate and blood pressure. Definitely lower blood triglycerides in individuals with high levels of these compounds. The increase in LDL with taking too many omega-3 pills may not be helpful. ALA may be just as important as EPA & DHA, but not enough money has been spent answering this question.
Dermatology (EPA & DHA)	Psoriasis, skin cancer
Gastroenterology (EPA & DHA)	Colorectal cancer, inflammatory bowel disease (Crohn's & ulcerative colitis)
Immunology/Infectious Disease/ Nephrology (EPA & DHA)	Allergies, asthma, hepatitis, IgA Nephropathy, lung function
Liver Disease (EPA & DHA)	Fatty liver and given with hepatitis C conventional treatment
Metabolic syndrome (EPA & DHA) (issues of high insulin or blood sugar levels, lots of belly fat, higher blood pressure & a low HDL & high triglycerides)	Omega-3 fatty acids may not only improve insulin sensitivity and lower triglycerides, but they also may help increase good cholesterol or HDL in some cases. They may help in weight reduction when taken in smaller amounts, but in large amounts they may cause weight gain.

Neurology (EPA & DHA)	Alzheimer's disease (especially DHA), dementia, autism (reduced hyperactivity in one clinical trial), ADHD …
Ob-Gyn/Pediatrics (ALA, EPA & DHA) Note: Women should supplement with about 300–600 mg of a total combination omega-3 fatty acids pill (ALA, EPA & DHA) during and after pregnancy.	Maternal & child health, cognitive (improved IQ) and visual impact in newborns & adolescents; improves gestation length, size, and potentially a variety of other outcomes such as post-partum depression.
Oncology (EPA & DHA)	Breast cancer, cachexia (reduces weight loss) if taking large amounts, colorectal cancer, endometrial cancer, leukemia, melanoma, ovarian cancer, pancreatic cancer, prostate cancer, renal cell cancer
Ophthalmology (EPA & DHA)	Macular degeneration, retinitis pigmentosa
Orthopedics (EPA & DHA)	Osteoporosis/fracture, inflammatory/ joint conditions (arthritis)
Psychiatry (EPA & DHA)	Depression, bipolar disorder, schizophrenia, ADHD Experts agree that DHA by itself does not impact depression, but that a combination of omega-3 (EPA & DHA) is best.
Rheumatology (EPA & DHA)	Rheumatoid arthritis, osteoarthritis, osteoporosis
Surgery (EPA & DHA)	Improve post-operative healing & other outcomes, but may also cause unwanted blood thinning if supplements taken preoperatively.
Urology (EPA & DHA)	Prostate cancer, prostatitis, BPH (prostate enlargement)

General Conclusions and Concerns

All of the omega-3 fatty acids alone and in combination need much more research before we can endorse a specific type and source, but get *all* 3 or at least 2 of 3 omega-3s (EPA & DHA) from your pill!

Omega-3 fatty acid pills look great for some people diagnosed with certain conditions or in pregnancy, but for people who are not carrying a child or those who are perfectly healthy, we are not sure of the impact of omega-3 compounds from pills, but this is being tested right now in large clinical trials. Most people need to consume more omega-3 fatty acids, but economics and education will help to reduce this problem because omega-3 compounds are now being added to many foods. Fish and omega-3 from fish and plant sources should be encouraged because these sources contain other healthy compounds, such as selenium and vitamin D.

The best recommendations for fish and fish oil pills are mostly from the American Heart Association (AHA) www.americanheart. org. They basically say two servings a week of oily, healthy fish and not more than about one pill a day (but up to 1,000 mg) of fish oil in those with documented heart disease. If there is a good reason, such as high triglycerides, depression, or arthritis, the recommended dosage increases to about 2–4 grams per day. *All high-dose conditions need to be worked out between you and your doctor to make sure the benefits outweigh the risks.*

So, eat a variety of oily fish about twice a week to get your EPA and DHA, and also try to consume a variety of vegetable oils (such as canola oil), nuts (such as walnuts), and seeds (flaxseed, for example) in order to get your ALA omega-3 fatty acids. Talk to your doctor about taking one or more fish oil pills a day for anything from depression to heart health or to relieve symptoms of osteoarthritis!

Dr. Moyad, I follow all your steps and am healthy—do I need to take a fish oil pill?

Whether or not to take just one fish oil pill per day if you are completely healthy and there is nothing wrong at all with you needs to be discussed with your doctor. Most fish oil pill takers are in this category, and we are not sure if this reduces the risk of any cardiac condition. We think it still helps you, but we are not sure. Keep in mind that in this group of individuals the risk of heart disease is so low that it will be difficult to ever have a clear answer! For healthy pregnant women and children or for those who do not eat any healthy fish, this group could see an enormous benefit, but again one to two pills a day is generally enough!

Dr. Moyad, are there side effects to taking fish oil?

Enteric coated fish oil pills can reduce the aftertaste and stomach upset, but whether or not these pills work as well as the regular fish oil pills remains to be seen. There are five key side effects with fish oil supplements that everyone should understand to some degree.

Measurement or Side Effect	Up to 1 gram a day of fish oil pills	1 to 3 grams a day of fish oil pills	More than 3 grams a day of fish oil pills
Bleeding or bruising	Very low risk	Very low risk	Low to moderate risk
Blood sugar levels increase, especially in diabetic patients	Very low risk	Low risk	Moderate risk
Cholesterol changes (LDL increases usually in individuals taking many grams because of high triglycerides)*	Very low risk	Moderate risk	Moderate to high risk
Fishy aftertaste (to reduce, use enteric coated, store pills in refrigerator or freezer, or take at night)	Low risk	Moderate risk	High risk
Stomach upset (to reduce, use enteric coated variety or take with food)	Very low risk	Low to moderate risk	Moderate risk

*Some argue that the increase in LDL is not a concern because fish oil may actually create larger LDL particles, which are not as dangerous.

Keep in mind that one of the most common side effects, pain reduction, with fish oil is really not a side effect. Patients report a decrease in back or arthritic pain because of the *anti-inflammatory* effects of omega-3 or fish oil. Again, mercury is not a concern in most fish oil capsules because the mercury (actually methylmercury, the toxic form) is water-soluble and not oil-soluble. When the oil is removed from the fish, the mercury, cadmium, lead, and other heavy metals stay behind and do not go into the pill. The other pollutants (many others are oil-soluble) are not an issue either because most pills come from the muscle of the fish and not the liver of the fish, where certain compounds can concentrate.

If you do not want to take a fish oil pill or an omega-3 enriched egg, there is another vegetarian/vegan option—micro-algae based omega-3 supplements. However, this should be a last resort because they usually contain one omega-3 (DHA).

Finally, always be sensitive to the "Moyad Add-Back Phenomenon," which means that you should always pick the lowest effective dose because while you are sleeping, popular and money-making nutrients are being added to your diet every day without getting your attention. Next year there will be close to 1,000 foods that have omega-3 added to them, and the current list of omega-3 enriched products continues to grow, such as milk, cereal, eggs, and margarine. So a deficiency today could be a situation of excess tomorrow!

**Please remember: Heart Healthy = All Healthy
and Heart Unhealthy = All Unhealthy!**

Multivitamins

| Dr. B.S.

"The human body needs several to many multivitamin pills a day, especially if you exercise a lot! Men and women need large doses of antioxidants in their multivitamins, but their needs are slightly different, so that is why I/we created two different multivitamin formulations ... one for the needs of a man and one for the needs of a woman."

| Dr. Moyad's No B.S.

"Whatever! Preliminary research suggests that multivitamins taken in very large quantities may potentially increase the risk of advanced and fatal cancers, such as prostate cancer. Taking one pill a day of a low-dose and cheap multivitamin may be very beneficial, but most men need to take a women's or children's multivitamin because they are based on science and not testosterone! A woman's one-pill-a-day multivitamin, with no iron and low to moderate amounts of other ingredients and larger amounts of calcium and vitamin D, is perfect for a man! Women who have not reached menopause need a multivitamin with iron, but women who have reached menopause do not necessarily need the extra iron, but again you and your doctor can make the best decision.

Yet another study came out recently (NIH-AARP study) that suggests that less is more when it comes to a variety of dietary supplement dosages. I have always been concerned that the average multivitamin continues to provide larger and larger quantities of antioxidants. The average multivitamin is getting so large that soon you will have to roll it into a truck to get it to your house. I found a best-selling multivitamin from 25 years ago recently. It only instructed the buyer to take one pill a day, and it had 10 vitamins and minerals. Take a look.

Ingredient	Popular Multivitamin Sold circa 1980s	Popular Multivitamin Sold Today
Vitamin A	5000 IU	5000 IU
Vitamin D	400 IU	400 IU
Vitamin E	15 IU	33 IU
Vitamin C	60 mg	60 mg
Folic acid	400 mcg	400 mcg
Vitamin B1 (thiamine)	1.5 mg	4.5 mg
Vitamin B2 (riboflavin)	1.7 mg	3.4 mg
Niacin	20 mg	20 mg
Vitamin B6	2 mg	6 mg
Vitamin B12	6 mcg	25 mcg
Vitamin K		20 mcg
Biotin		30 mcg
Pantothenic acid		15 mg
Calcium		400 mg
Chloride		90 mg
Iodine		150 mcg
Magnesium		50 mg
Potassium		100 mg
Zinc		22.5 mg
Selenium		20 mcg
Copper		2 mg

Ingredient	Popular Multivitamin Sold circa 1980s	Popular Multivitamin Sold Today
Manganese		4 mg
Iron		20 mg
Boron		150 mcg
Chromium		180 mcg
Molybdenum		90 mcg
Nickel		5 mcg
Silicon		5 mg
Tin		10 mcg
Vanadium		10 mcg
Lycopene		50 mcg
Ginkgo biloba		120 mg
Ginseng		10 mg
Other herbs		Variety of doses
Caffeine		Variety of doses

Men who were free of cancer who participated in the National In-stitutes of Health (NIH)-AARP Diet and Health Study were evaluated. Basically, this study selected from the 3.5 million AARP members, 50–71 years old, who lived in one of six states or two metropolitan areas. These men were fairly healthy. About 5 percent of the men in this study were heavy users of multivitamins (a total of 13,854 men), and overall multivitamins were the most commonly ingested supple-ments (51 percent), followed by vitamin C (40 percent), vitamin E (37 percent), and calcium (22 percent).

Overall, no association was found between the use of multivita-mins and the overall risk for localized prostate cancer. However, an increased risk of advanced and fatal prostate cancer was found for the men reporting an intake of more than seven multivitamin pills a week. This troubling correlation was found to be even stronger for men who were heavy users of multivitamins and those who also had a family history of prostate cancer and/or who took higher amounts of additional individual supplements, including beta-carotene, sele-nium, and zinc. Another concern found in the study, but apparently not statistically significant, was that men in the high-use multivitamin group consumed almost 100 calories more per day than the other men in the lower supplement intake groups.

However, perhaps the best news from this study that did not receive much attention was for men taking one multivitamin a day, which represented the largest numbers of men followed in the study. Men had a 10 to 20 percent reduced risk of fatal prostate cancer in this group, and they were the only group to demonstrate a lower significant risk of dying from prostate cancer in this study. Everything in moderation.

Now let me tell you about the mini-multivitamin study that no one knows about, but everyone should know about now! The SU.VI. MAX Study was a randomized, double-blind, placebo-controlled primary prevention trial (participants were completely healthy at the start of the trial) that was recently published and *is one of the most powerful studies of my lifetime to show that less is more with your multivitamin.* A total of 13,017 French adults (7,876 women aged 35–60 years, average age 46 to 47, and 5,141 men aged 45–60 years, average age 51 years) were included in this study. This is the healthiest group of people I have ever come across in all my medical research experience (the average person was of normal weight, and 85 percent of the participants were non-smokers ...). All of the individuals took either a placebo or a daily capsule that consisted of 120 mg of vitamin C, 30 mg of vitamin E, 6 mg of beta-carotene, 100 mcg of selenium, and 20 mg of zinc.

These individuals were then followed for 7.5 years! Nothing bad or good happened in the group as a whole, but when they looked at the men in this study a difference or an impact occurred. There was a 31 percent reduction in the risk of being diagnosed with cancer in the men only, and a 37 percent reduction in the risk of dying from any cause in men! Wow! It seems that taking a low-dose multivitamin may have had a profound effect or benefit for men. The researchers from this study believe that men benefited because they had lower levels of antioxidants (especially vitamin C and beta-carotene) in their blood at the beginning of the study compared to the women. The women were very healthy in this study.

Finally, a follow-up to this study (8.8 to 9 years later) found that this multivitamin reduced the risk of prostate cancer by 48 percent in men with a low PSA (less than 3), but in men with a higher PSA, a multivitamin may have been associated with a higher risk of getting prostate cancer. In other words, if a man has an elevated PSA he should be careful about taking dietary supplements to reduce risk and should talk to his doctor first. This multivitamin did not impact PSA or insulin-like growth factor (IGF) levels, suggesting that risk was affected by other methods. It was also interesting in this study that older men (the average age of men was 51 years), more obese men, and men with higher PSA levels had a significantly increased risk for prostate cancer. No individuals discontinued the study because of side effects from the multivitamin. One limitation in this study was that no information was collected on family history of prostate cancer.

So my advice is simple (until we get more research):

- Men of all ages should basically consume one pill a day (maximum) of a women's or children's low-dose multivitamin with low or no iron, because they are usually high in two ingredients, calcium and vitamin D, which is exactly more of what men and women need! The rest of the ingredients should be in moderate to low and safe levels (not higher than the recommended daily allowance or the percent daily value).
- Pre-menopausal women should consume a one-pill-a-day women's multivitamin that has iron (around 20 mg), and only higher doses of calcium and vitamin D (same as the men above but with iron), and at least the recommended daily dose of B vitamins, including 400 mcg a day of folic acid.
- Post-menopausal women should consume the same low-dose women's multivitamin above (that the men take) that has no iron and only higher amounts of calcium and vitamin D.

**Please remember: Heart Healthy = All Healthy
and Heart Unhealthy = All Unhealthy!**

Vitamin C

Vitamin C is perhaps the most researched nutrient/product in the world and *the one taken by the most patients and health-care professionals around the world*. But does it work?

| Dr. B.S.

"Vitamin C is not needed in a higher dose than the recommended daily allowance of 60 mg per day because the recommended daily allowance is enough to cure scurvy!"

| Dr. Moyad's No B.S.

"Whatever! While it is true that 60 mg per day is enough to stave off scurvy, we should examine vitamin C again for what the chronic disease prevention clinical trials have taught us."

Let's review some medical conditions and the potential impact on these conditions with normal blood levels of vitamin C from taking a vitamin C supplement as opposed to getting it from just fruits and vegetables. You might find some of the results startling. The most comprehensive research in the field has been done for calcium ascorbate (Ester-C®), as compared to any other form of vitamin C. The safety record of vitamin C supplements is outstanding, and there is enough research done with calcium ascorbate to fill a library. Lets's take a look at the sum of the evidence.

The research considered here is not associated with eating more fruits and vegetables, but actually taking a pill in a dosage of at least 500 mg a day (the most tested and safe clinical trial dose). By eating five servings a day of fruits and vegetables that especially contain higher amounts of vitamin C, you will be able to absorb about 200 mg of vitamin C. However, most people consume fewer than five servings a day, so trying to achieve 500 mg a day through dietary vitamin C does not work for most people.

Allergies (seasonal)/Asthma

Recent preliminary clinical studies have suggested that vitamin C can lower the needed dosage of conventional medication, such as steroid use in children, especially in adults with asthma-like symptoms when used at 500 to 1000 mg (1 gram) a day and over several months. Vitamin C has the potential to reduce the risk and impact of allergies or asthma, perhaps due to its ability to lower histamine blood levels. Histamine is the major culprit for sneezing, wheezing, runny noses, and watery eyes. Antihistamine medications work to relieve the symptoms caused by histamine, but research is showing that vitamin C can give some relief without some of the negative effects of antihistamines, such as drowsiness. Higher doses of vitamin C are being studied now in individuals who have exercise-induced asthma or airway constriction, and the preliminary results suggest a benefit in reducing this problem.

Arthritis

In a random trial of 2 grams of calcium ascorbate versus placebo, patients reported significant reduction in the pain associated with osteoarthritis of the knee. Additional studies are needed to substantiate the findings from this first clinical trial.

Bone Fractures

A major trial of over 300 patients, recently published in the *Journal of Bone and Joint Surgery*, studied varying doses of vitamin C and found that these supplements reduced some of the complications or problems associated with casts applied after suffering a bone fracture. The most effective dosage in the trial was 500 mg/day, which reduced the risk of associated problems by 59 percent. Particularly in wrist fractures, vitamin C has been shown to reduce the risk of at least four of the five problems associated with bone fracture and cast—pain, difference in skin color, tissue swelling (edema), skin temperature difference, or limited range of motion of the area.

Bone Health

Studies currently underway have seen higher vitamin D levels in patients with higher blood levels of vitamin C. Since vitamin C helps to maintain the primary infrastructure of tissue and bone (collagen), could higher blood levels of vitamin C be associated with less bone loss? I do believe that vitamin C has some impact on maintaining bone health.

Cancer

The first major trial that I discussed earlier in the multivitamin section was the SU.VI.MAX trial, which has shown a reduced risk of cancer for men with higher blood levels of vitamin C (1.1 to 1.3 mg/dL). Vitamin C at 500 mg/day (versus placebo) is currently part of one of the largest cancer prevention trials in human history—PHS II (Physicians' Health Study II). After the first major trial, I began to believe that perhaps there could be some protective impact with higher blood levels. Future trials will provide more clarity. Intravenous vitamin C also looks interesting, but it bothers me that I have seen all sorts of ridiculous cure claims. I think it is fair to say that, at this point, we don't have a clear idea if vitamin C is good, bad, or without impact on cancer.

Cardiovascular Health

Vitamin C is associated with a lower risk of cardiovascular disease, especially stroke, and the most common dosage in clinical trials was 500 mg/day. Also, higher blood levels of vitamin C tend to be associated with better health, such as not smoking, moderate alcohol intake, less belly fat, etc., so this is why I am beginning to think that more doctors need to offer vitamin C blood testing every so often to patients just to see how they are doing. Vitamin C is associated with a healthy lifestyle, but is it the lifestyle, the supplement, or both that are contributing to the lower risk of heart disease?

Colds/Influenza/Pneumonia

One of the largest meta-analyses ever of vitamin C over the past thirty years showed that getting about 500 mg/day was associated with a lower risk of getting pneumonia and a greater chance of surviving or recovering from pneumonia when vitamin C was used along with conventional prescription medication. Do I think it reduces the risk of cold and flu? I do, but it doesn't matter what I think about this because at least it seems to reduce the risk of lung infection and pneumonia that can develop from a simple infection. Pneumonia is a major killer.

Dental Health

Tooth or dental health and gum health rely on vitamin C to keep the mouth and teeth tightly woven in place (with collagen) and free of disease. Now you know why the initial claim to fame of this vitamin was for tooth and dental health (to prevent scurvy).

Energy Levels/Reduce Fatigue

Carnitine, which is made by every cell of the human body, cannot be made without vitamin C! Carnitine takes fuel or fatty acids into every cell to make energy, and that is why researchers are studying carnitine to reduce fatigue and improve energy levels in people with many diseases (e.g., cancer and multiple sclerosis). Vitamin C sacrifices itself in the human body so that carnitine can be produced. However, there is no point to increasing carnitine (sold as a nutritional supplement) unless a person is increasing his or her blood level of vitamin C.

Exercise

Researchers are looking into the possibility of vitamin C supplementation to reduce muscle fatigue and soreness after aerobic exercise and weight lifting. One very good weight-lifting study found that vitamin C after a workout reduced muscle fatigue and blood markers of muscle fatigue so that lifting a few days later was easier to do. There are already a few clinical studies utilizing about 500 to 1000 mg/day. It would make sense because of how vitamin C improves carnitine levels in the body, but I would like to see more research in this area. Extreme exercise can deplete vitamin C levels quickly, and this is why even in the studies of cold prevention there is very good agreement that vitamin C can reduce infections in individuals who exercise daily.

Eye Health

Five hundred milligrams of vitamin C is part of the standard dosage of a combination eye health supplement (along with 400 mg of vitamin E, 15 mg of beta-carotene, 80 mg of zinc oxide, and 2 mg of cupric oxide) that has been associated with a reduced risk of vision loss from macular degeneration (the number-one cause of blindness in the United States). This was tested in one of the largest government-funded studies in human history (AREDS). However, the only nutrient from this study that has been shown to be safe without any serious catch has been vitamin C. Vitamin C is also being studied in the area of cataract prevention and to see if it improves the recovery time from LASIK surgery if vitamin C is taken several days before or after surgery, because many doctors have been using it for years for this purpose.

Fertility/Infertility/Birth Control

Vitamin C is associated with a higher potential sperm count or ability of sperm to reach its destination. Much of the fluid added to sperm during its path has very high levels of vitamin C. Some clinical studies have used very large amounts of vitamin C in men, such as a study of 1,000 mg two times a day, that improved sperm count, motility, and morphology. These studies need to be longer in order to determine if vitamin C can actually and significantly improve the chances of pregnancy in those couples who have had a difficult time getting pregnant.

Immunology/Immune Boost/Infectious Disease

The results of a recent large study of over 400 blood samples was presented to determine if vitamin C was the fuel used by immune cells to generate an immune boost or a better immune response. This result had been found in the past. Researchers found that normal or higher vitamin C blood levels were associated with stronger immune responses, but they also found that calcium ascorbate was kept inside the immune cells to a greater degree compared to vitamin C, despite patients having similar blood levels of vitamin C. In other words, it is possible that because calcium ascorbate was easier to take (it is non-acidic) and/or contains metabolites of vitamin C, it may provide a greater immune response over a 24-hour period. Regardless, immune cells or leukocytes in general contain 10–50 times the concentration of vitamin C compared to general blood levels.

Maternal/Child Health

Vitamin C has one of its most critical roles in the area of pregnancy and maternal and child health by increasing the absorption of iron from food and supplements, and reducing the risk of anemia in pregnancy. Vitamin C requirements increase during pregnancy. This is why the number-one-selling prescription prenatal vitamin (PrimaCare® One) has calcium ascorbate in every box, and so does the top-selling individualized prescription iron supplement (Repliva®) for iron-deficient women. The most critical components in prenatal vitamins (prescription or not) are the B vitamins like folic acid to reduce the risk of birth defects, but the next most critical components would have to be vitamin C and vitamin D. Pregnant women also have a higher chance of suffering from acid reflux because hormone changes in pregnancy make it easier for acid to go back up the esophagus. For this reason, I suggest that pregnant women need to take a nonacidic form of vitamin C that has been tested.

Medical Procedures

Vitamin C is being seriously considered as a potential way to reduce the side effects or risk of kidney, heart, or other organ damage from medical contrast dyes used in visualizing anatomy in many hospital procedures. Some recent clinical trials have had patients take vitamin C before the imaging test was done, and it seemed to reduce the toxicity of these contrast dyes. Stay tuned!

Mental Health

Researchers know for certain that vitamin C is involved in several pathways that improve neurotransmitter levels in the brain and the rest of the body. Consequently, there is now enormous interest in the area of vitamin C and mental health. The more intense area of study is with depression, as there seems to be greater nutritional deficiencies in persons with this disease.

Skin Health/Anti-aging

Vitamin C, compared to any other nutrient, was associated with the greatest reductions in the signs of aging, skin damage, wrinkles, and skin atrophy (thinning) in one of the largest government studies (the National Health and Nutrition Examination Survey) in human history to look at this issue. I wonder why everyone is now putting vitamin C in all the skin creams and antiaging lotions! In reality, this was another situation where vitamin C supplements were not necessarily the primary reason; vitamin C levels and intake were instead associated with a healthier lifestyle such as more physical activity. Vitamin C is involved in collagen production and the regeneration process of skin and in wound repair.

Sleep

Vitamin C may reduce the negative impact of not getting enough sleep by maintaining blood flow and immune defenses. This has already been demonstrated in some clinical studies. Now, the solution is to get more sleep, of course, but during those times that you know there will be some serious deprivation, I suggest more vitamin C.

Smoking

Smoking is famous for a serious deficiency in one nutrient, and that is vitamin C. In fact, the vitamin C requirements for smokers are the highest for any group. However, this discussion is silly and mundane because the issue with smokers is that they need to stop smoking or using lethal tobacco products now. I do not want to recommend higher intakes of vitamin C to a smoker, but rather I want to recommend higher intakes to ex-smokers because they also have nutrient issues for years after quitting.

Stomach/Intestinal Health and Reflux Disease

In clinical trials patients have preferred nonacidic calcium ascorbate over regular vitamin C tablets in order to reduce acid reflux. Acid reflux medication is one of the most commonly prescribed drugs. When I consult with patients, I like them to take calcium ascorbate but at the same time reduce their intake of the acid reflux medication by following the Moyad lifestyle steps in this book. Vitamin C is also being studied along with the combination of acid reflux medication and antibiotics (called triple therapy) to eliminate the bacteria (H. pylori) that causes most ulcers and some stomach and intestinal cancers.

Stress (Mental and Physical)

In the results of recent studies, authors have reported that vitamin C supplements, even at low dosages (500 mg/day), are associated with significantly lower rates of infection in people *under stress of a variety of types* (exercise, temperature). Some of the most negative studies of vitamin C for colds actually were some of the most positive in my opinion as to why we should continue the research in this area and in the area of stress.

Surgery

Vitamin C improves wound healing, but does this mean you should take vitamin C after a surgical procedure? I am leaving this discussion to you and your surgeon who knows your case.

Urologic/Kidney Health

Calcium ascorbate has been associated with lower oxalate levels compared to vitamin C, so it may be associated with a lower risk of kidney stones. Researchers are testing this right now, because legitimate concerns about megadosing with vitamin C supplements exist. I do not believe in megadosing; the evidence is weak, and the only real potential side effect is a higher risk of kidney stones. A previous clinical study showed a reduced risk of kidney stones with calcium ascorbate, but I refuse to believe in this benefit until it is clinically researched one more time. Researchers are doing this now, and I look forward to seeing if this is the case.

Dr. Moyad, I want to keep it simple, but I need to still ask you about those Airborne®-like supplements and generic products from the tablets to the fizzy kind of options?

Do you ever notice that as life gets more complicated, preventive medicine gets more simplistic? These products have sold well in the past and are a mixture of multiple amounts of vitamins, minerals, herbal products, and a great marketing story. These products do not have any good human clinical research, but that does not mean they are worthless. I find it interesting that one of the largest ingredients in these products is *vitamin C with about 1,000 mg per tablet*! Save your money and just buy vitamin C or Ester-C.

Dr. Moyad, how about the new exotic berry products that are touted to prevent all sorts of diseases?

Goji berry is an interesting story. The bitter berry is indigenous to the lush valleys of the Himalayan Mountains. They taste like a cross between olives and cranberries, and the claims have been amazing! Are they the fountain of youth? Apparently, they have 15 times the antioxidant power of other fruit and 500 times more vitamin C by weight than fresh oranges, six times more amino acids than bee pollen, and more iron than spinach! The claims are amazing because you name it and some person or business has claimed that it may prevent or cure it, and of course it is not cheap! What this berry needs is some of the large amount of money being made on it to fund a study so that the research can support the hype. Again, I find it interesting that what we certainly know is that it contains a high concentration of a vitamin C–like compound.

Conclusions

Think of all the tests, lifestyle changes, and pills that were covered in this book. It is enough already to keep you busy the rest of your life with your doctor and make your head spin for a while! So, in my opinion, it is ridiculous to consider taking any other pills right now until you review the contents of this section again and again. Life is worth enjoying and living, so the next time you read some of the more B.S. health magazines or books, try to guess how many pills they want you to take after reading it from cover to cover. The last magazine I read had me taking 38 pills from just one issue! If they say you are supposed to take more pills than are discussed in this section of the book and you are perfectly healthy, perhaps it is time for a little reflection.

This now brings me to the *most serious commentary in the entire book*, which is the following:

"Surveys suggest that fewer than 5 percent of consumers even know or follow just some of the information that you have just covered. From my experience, I would say it is *less than 1 percent*. I would include many health-care professionals in this estimate. This is nobody's fault, but focusing on consumer and preventive health should be a medical specialty. However, it is not!"

You should never allow yourself to follow lifestyle, supplement, or preventive advice from a doctor or another health-care professional who does not do this job full-time or at least does not make it his or her primary calling in life! It seems so easy to just throw out advice in the area, because what possible harm could result from some healthy advice? In my experience, the harm that I have seen is as serious as a botched surgery! How can that be? I have witnessed hundreds, probably now thousands of men and women who spent their golden years and even their retirement money on health practices and advice that were not only worthless but occupied so much of their time that they had a low quality of life.

This is the biggest danger and arrogance of bogus preventive medicine! The user has the potential to be the ultimate Monday morning quarterback, but with far more serious consequences than any athletic outcome. It seems benign on the outside, but in reality it can be as damaging as amputating the wrong leg during surgery. The difference is that the surgical outcome is tangible, and one knows almost immediately if things went right or wrong. However, with lifestyle or preventive medical advice, it can be years and years before one realizes the damage that has been done.

I was in a restaurant the other day, and a guy who recognized me from a community lecture brought a very popular book with him, placed it on my table, and essentially said, "Dr. B.S.'s book tells me I *have* to go out and take this preventive pill every day to increase my life expectancy." I said that is B.S., and then I asked him if I could do surgery on him immediately or at least by tomorrow? He laughed and said, "But you are not a surgeon and are not qualified to do that procedure, and I do not think I need that procedure because I do not qualify for it, do I? I mean, there has to be some individualized criterion or threshold or standard for whether or not someone needs this procedure." And I said, "Good for you; you are absolutely 100 percent right. Now go out and apply those same principles to the ridiculous preventive health advice that you received from that book and any other B.S. source that happens to cross your path. Remember if you *qualify* for a pill it can save your life, but if you do not qualify for it and recklessly just take it without any risk assessment, it can *wreck your life.*"

**Remember: Heart Healthy = All Healthy
and Heart Unhealthy = All Unhealthy.**

Moyad Immune Quotient (MIQ)

(your final moderate, practical and probability-based no B.S. health exam to really see how you are doing right now)

What Is Your MIQ?
Circle the answer to each question.

1. **I currently smoke.**

    A. Yes (–10 points, yes, that is a minus)
    B. No (0 points)

2. **What is your LDL (bad cholesterol) untreated or treated with medication?**

    A. Less than 100 mg/dl or 2.59 mmol/L (4 points)
    B. 100–129 mg/dl or 2.59–3.34 mmol/L (3 points)
    C. 130–159 mg/dl or 3.37–4.12 mmol/L (2 points)
    D. 160–189 mg/dl or 4.14–4.90 mmol/L (1 point)
    E. 190 mg/dl or 4.92 mmol/L and above (0 points)
    F. Do not know the answer (–1 point)

3. **What is your HDL (good cholesterol) untreated or treated with medication?**

    A. 60 mg/dl or 1.55 mmol/L and above (4 points)
    B. 50–59 mg/dl or 1.29–1.53 mmol/L (3 points)
    C. 40–49 mg/dl or 1.04–1.27 mmol/L (2 points)
    D. 35–39 mg/dl or 0.91–1.01 mmol/L (1 point)
    E. Below 35 mg/dl or 0.91 mmol/L (0 points)
    F. Do not know the answer (–1 point)

4. **What is your triglyceride number untreated or treated with medication?**

    A. Less than 100 mg/dl or 1.13 mmol/L (4 points)
    B. 100–149 mg/dl or 1.13–1.68 mmol/L (3 points)
    C. 150–199 mg/dl or 1.70–2.25 mmol/L (2 points)
    D. 200–499 mg/dl or 2.26–5.64 mmol/L (1 point)
    E. 500 mg/dl or 5.65 mmol/L and above (0 points)
    F. Do not know the answer (–1 point)

5. **My hs-CRP (high sensitivity C-Reactive protein) blood level is:**

    A. Normal (2 points)
    B. Abnormal (1 points)
    C. I don't know/have not had this tested (–1)

6. **My fasting blood glucose level is:**

   A. Normal (2 points)
   B. Abnormal (1 points)
   C. I don't know/have not had this tested (−1)

7. **My blood pressure untreated or treated is:**

   A. Less than 120/80 mmHg (4 points)
   B. 120–139 and/or 80–89 mmHg(3 points)
   C. 140 or higher and/or 90 mmHg or higher (2 points)
   D. Do not know (1 point)

8. **Framingham Risk Score**

   A. My Framingham Risk Score number is _____ and I will take it to my doctor. (4 points)
   B. I do not know what this is or how to calculate the number (0 points)

9. **My weight is _____ and my height is _____; my body mass index (BMI) is _____; my waist circumference (WC) is _____; and my waist-to-hip ratio (WHR) is _____.**

   A. Filled in all 5 blanks above (4 points)
   B. Filled in 4 of the 5 blanks above (3 points)
   C. Filled in 3 of the 5 blanks above (2 points)
   D. Filled in 2 of the 5 blanks above (1 point)
   E. Do not know any of these numbers (0 points)

10. **My family health history tree**

    A. Yes, I have reviewed my complete family health history tree and found that I have a higher risk of _____. (4 points)
    B. No, I have not reviewed my complete family health history tree. (0 points)
    C. Do you sell the seeds for such a tree, Dr. Moyad? (−100 points)

11. **Based on your health history and family health history, what screening tests do you need in the next year?**

    A. _____ (4 points for just coming up with an answer that can be discussed with your doctor at your next visit)
    B. I do not know. (0 points)

12. **What are you going to do for your spirituality project in the next 12 months?**

    A. _____ (4 points for just coming up with an answer that you may consider doing over the next several months)
    B. What do you mean by spirituality project? (0 points)

13. **Aerobic exercise and/or weight-lifting/resistance exercise**

    A. I exercise an average of 30 minutes a day and lift weights/resistance exercise 2 to 3 times a week? (4 points)
    B. I only exercise an average of 30 minutes a day, but I do not lift weights/resistance exercise on a regular basis. (3 points)
    C. I only lift weights/resistance exercise regularly, but do not do regular aerobic exercise (2 points).
    D. I do not exercise or lift weight/resistance exercise regularly (1 point).
    E. I do not have any time to exercise or lift weights/resistance exercise (0 points)

14. **3,500 calories (14,644 KJ) is equivalent to:**

    A. 0.25 pounds or 0.125 kilograms (4 points)
    B. 0.50 pounds or 0.25 kilograms (3 points)
    C. 0.75 pounds or 0.33 kilograms (2 points)
    D. 1 pound or 0.5 kilograms (1 point)
    E. I have no idea (0 points)

15. **What does the answer from question 14 really mean in the real world?**

    A. Losing weight is really really hard to do. (4 points)
    B. Losing weight is hard to do. (3 points)
    C. Losing weight is moderately hard to do. (2 points)
    D. Losing weight is easy. (1 point)
    E. Losing weight is hard or easy depending on your genetics. (0 points)

16. **Two types of "healthy" dietary fats are _____ & _____.**

    A. Monounsaturated and polyunsaturated fat (4 points)
    B. Monounsaturated and trans fat (3 points)
    C. Polyunsaturated and trans fat (2 points)
    D. Saturated and trans fat (1 point)

E. All dietary fat is unhealthy (0 points)

17. **How many servings of alcohol do you drink a day?**
(1 serving is 12 ounces of beer, 4–6 ounces of wine, or 1.5 ounces of hard liquor)

   A. If female 1 or less servings/day & if male 2 or less servings/day (4 points)
   B. If female 2 or less servings/day & if male 3 or less servings/day (2 points)
   C. Any other answer (0 points)

18. **How much fiber do you get in your diet per day?**

   A. 20–30 grams a day and mostly insoluble fiber (4 points)
   B. 20–30 grams a day and mostly soluble fiber (3 points)
   C. 10–20 grams a day and mostly insoluble fiber (2 points)
   D. 10–20 grams a day and mostly soluble fiber (1 point)
   E. Less than 10 grams a day (0 points)
   F. I do not know (–1 point)

19. **I get my omega-3 fatty acids mostly from eating:**

   A. Plant sources and 2–3 servings/week of non-fried small- to medium-size oily fish such as anchovies, mackerel, salmon, sardines … (4 points)
   B. Plant sources and 1–2 servings/week of non-fried small- to medium-size oily fish such as anchovies, mackerel, salmon, sardines … (3 points)
   C. Plant sources and 0–1 servings/week of non-fried small- to medium-size oily fish such as anchovies, mackerel, salmon, sardines … (2 points)
   D. I just take a fish oil pill (1 point)
   E. I do not eat fish or a take a fish oil pill (0 points)

20. **How many servings of fruits and vegetables do you eat per day?**

   A. More than 1 serving a day (4 points)
   B. Less than 1 serving a day (3 points)
   C. A couple of servings a week (2 points)
   D. A couple of servings a month (1 point)
   E. I do not like fruits or vegetables (0 points)
   F. I only eat colorful fruits and veggies because they are the healthiest. (–1 point)

21. **I like fruits and vegetable juices that:**
    A. Taste good and have the lowest calories (4 points)
    B. Taste good regardless of calories (1 point)
    C. Regardless of taste, have the highest concentration of antioxidants (0 points)

22. **Nuts that have the highest ratio of _____ are the healthiest.**
    A. Monounsaturated + polyunsaturated to saturated fat (4 points)
    B. Monounsaturated to saturated fat (3 points)
    C. Polyunsaturated to saturated fat (2 points)
    D. Saturated to monounsaturated + polyunsaturated (1 point)
    E. Trans fat to saturated fat (0 points)

23. **Cooking oils that have the highest ratio of _____ are the healthiest.**
    A. Monounsaturated + polyunsaturated: saturated fat (4 points)
    B. Monounsaturated to saturated fat (3 points)
    C. Polyunsaturated to saturated fat (2 points)
    D. Saturated to monounsaturated + polyunsaturated (1 point)
    E. Trans fat to saturated fat (0 points)

24. **I eat _____ of cheap dietary sources of plant estrogens (flax, sesame seed, or soy) a week and not just for the plant estrogen but for the fiber, omega-3 fatty acids, and low amount of calories.**
    A. Several servings (4 points)
    B. Hardly any servings (2 points)
    C. No servings (0 points)

25. **I like to have sex/make love with my partner at least:**
    A. Several times a week (1 point)
    B. Once a week (1 point)
    C. Once every 2 weeks or month (0 points)
    D. Not that often (0 points)
    E. I do not like to have sex with my partner. (−1 point)

26. I average about ___ hours of sleep per night.

    A. 7–8 hours (1 point)
    B. 5–6 hours (1 point)
    C. 3–4 hours (0 points)

27. I get ___ milligrams (mg) of sodium a day from food and beverages.

    A. 1,500 mg or less (1 point)
    B. 1,501 mg to 2,300 mg (1 point)
    C. 2,301 mg or more (0 points)

28. My mood level is in generally:

    A. Excellent, usually very happy (1 point)
    B. Very good, usually happy (1 point)
    C. Good, moderately happy (1 point)
    D. Indifferent, not really happy or sad (0 points)
    E. Bad (–1 point)

29. My vitamin D (25-OH vitamin D) blood level (taken in the fall or winter usually) is:

    A. Greater than 40 ng/ml or 100 nmol/L (4 points)
    B. 30–39 ng/ml or 75–99 nmol/L (2 points)
    C. Below 30 ng/ml or 75 nmol/L (0 points)
    D. I have not had a vitamin D blood test (–1 point)

30. I never take any pill without first figuring out with the doctor I trust the most if I personally *qualify for a pill,* and that includes prescription drugs and dietary supplements. (If *true,* give yourself 1 point). In other words, only after reviewing all my tests, family history, and after complete risk assessment and understanding of the latest and largest clinical trials paid for by the taxpayers will I then decide whether or not to take any pill. Even if I take a pill, I always reevaluate every year whether or not I still need to take this pill and/or the same dosage of this pill.

    A. All of the above is true (4 points)
    B. All of the above is partly true (1 point)
    C. The above information does not make sense to me (0 points)

Extra Credit Points

- I have talked to my employer about more exercise time, and now my work schedule revolves around my health. (1 point for Yes)
- I have purchased and used my own automated blood pressure device at home. (1 point for Yes)
- Women only–I have completed a Reynolds Risk Score on the computer, and my risk is _____%. (1 point)
- Men only—I understand that if I am married that I get a health benefit just by being married even though my wife may not, but I will never admit this fact to her. (1 point for accepting this statement as true)
- I now understand that less is more when it comes to my health and pills. (If this makes sense to you, give yourself 1 point. If it does not make sense, please go back and read Dr. Moyad's book again.)

Add your points: _____

Note: The following grades are given just like in school.

100+ = A+ (You need to write a book and give lectures and stop listening to me.)
90–99 = A (You are the woman! You are the man!)
80–89 = B (Doing well, but need some work to become the woman or man.)
70–79 = C (You are average and need to stay after school.)
60–69 = D (Have your parents sign this immediately.)
50–59 = E/F (Go see the principal right now, please.)

Oh, but wait! Please, I hope you have not read this book if you are more worried about having questions similar to the following answered rather than the more serious questions, such as "What could end my life in a moment?"

Someone has asked me the following questions at least once. They are included here because laughter is beneficial to your immune system.

- There are so many PIN numbers to memorize, Dr. Moyad. Would it help to take ginkgo biloba to memorize them all?

- Dr. Moyad, I need to know which one is better—farm-raised or wild salmon—because even though I don't eat much fish, it would help to know which is healthier. And is a Filet-O-Fish sandwich farm- or wild-raised?
- I hear dark chocolate and dark beer have more antioxidants, so do I have to throw out my regular chocolate bars and my favorite beer, Dr. Moyad? The other day when I was picking up a pack of smokes from the store, the person behind the counter was on the phone and telling someone about this new research on dark chocolate and beer, and I was like wow, I have to ask Dr. Moyad about this, so what do you think?
- Dr. Moyad, I read recently that 50 percent of men who use public restrooms do not wash their hands after using a toilet, but I ask you Dr. Moyad, what is more troubling—the fact that half of the men did not wash their hands or the fact that so-called well-educated researchers hid in a toilet stall with a hole drilled in the wall with a clipboard and pen to secretly observe men using a urinal to then see if they washed their hands? Which fact do you find more troubling?

Index